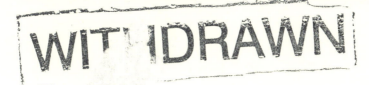

BEING MENTALLY ILL

Third Edition

BEING MENTALLY ILL
A Sociological Theory

(Third Edition)

Thomas J. Scheff

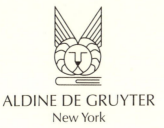

ALDINE DE GRUYTER
New York

About the Author

Thomas J. Scheff is Professor Emeritus of Sociology, University of California, Santa Barbara. He is author of *Emotions, the Social Bond, and Human Reality; Bloody Revenge; Catharsis in Healing, Ritual, and Drama;* and coauthor of *Emotions and Violence.*

ALDINE DE GRUYTER
A division of Walter de Gruyter, Inc.
200 Saw Mill River Road
Hawthorne, New York 10532

This publication is printed on acid free paper ⊖

Library of Congress Cataloging-in-Publication Data

Scheff, Thomas J.
 Being mentally ill : sociological theory / Thomas J. Scheff. — 3rd ed.
  p. cm.
 Includes bibliographical references and index.
 ISBN 0-202-30586-4 (cl. : alk. paper) — ISBN 0-202-30587-2 (pa. : alk. paper)
 1. Mental illness–Etiology—Social aspects. 2. Mental illness. 3. Social role. I. Title.

RC455 .S25 1999
362.2—dc21   99-045679

Manufactured in the United States of America
10 9 8 7 6 5 4 3 2 1

Contents

    The Origins of Residual Rule-Breaking   58
    Prevalence   63
    The Duration and Consequences
        of Residual Rule-Breaking   65

5   The Social Institution of Insanity   69

    Individual and Interpersonal Systems
        in Role-Playing   70
    Learning and Maintaining Role Imagery   74
    Normalization and Labeling   84
    Acceptance of the Deviant Role   86
    A Note on Feedback in
        Deviance-Amplifying Systems   94
    Conclusion   97

PART III   THE POWER OF THE PSYCHIATRIST

    Type 1 and Type 2 Errors   103
    Decision Rules in Medicine   104
    Basic Assumptions   106
    The "Sick Role"   108
    Implications for Research   110

7   Negotiating Reality:
    Notes on Power in the Assessment
    of Responsibility   115

    The Process of Negotiation   120
    A Contrasting Case   123
    Discussion   126
    Conclusion:
        Negotiation in Social Science Research   130

PART IV   THE EMOTIONAL/RELATIONAL WORLD

Preface

The first edition of this book (1966) presented a sociological theory of mental disorder. Seeing mental disorder from the point of view of a single discipline, the theory was one-dimensional. The second edition (1984), except for slight changes, continued in this same vein. Since that time there have been substantial advances in the biology, psychology, and even in the sociology of mental disorder. What is now most needed is an interdisciplinary approach, one that would integrate the disparate languages, viewpoints, and findings of the relevant disciplines. Such an integrated approach would be far greater than the sum of its parts, the separate disciplines. In human conduct, particularly, the vital processes seem to occur at interfaces, in the intersections of organic, psychological, and social systems.

To use E. O. Wilson's term (1998), what we want is "consilience," the interlocking of frameworks from the relevant disciplines. Although not using that word, I had proposed a similar interlocking for the social sciences (Scheff 1997) and illustrated what it would look like with several of my own studies. As Wilson indicates, many of the recent triumphs of the physical and life sciences have been based on the integration of the various disciplinary approaches.

As Wilson also indicates, there has been very little consilience among the behavioral and social sciences. Each of these disciplines goes its own way, ignoring the adjacent disciplines. Each emphasizes its own virtues, largely ignoring its weaknesses, as in the old song: "You got to accentuate the positive, eliminate the negative, tune in to the affirmative, don't mess with Mr. Inbetween." Contrary to the song, we must begin to mess with Mr. Inbetween.

Given the need for consilience, is there any point in resurrecting labeling theory, yet another one-dimensional approach to the complex problem of mental disorder? Before preparing this edition, I gave thought to this issue. My decision that the theory still had value was based on the following ideas. First, while waiting for consilient approaches to be developed, headway can still be made with one- or two-dimensional approaches. As will be proposed in Chapter 1, biopsychiatry, an integration of biology and psychiatry, seems to have made many worthwhile advances in the understanding and treatment of mental disorder. In the last twenty years, even one-dimensional studies of labeling of mental disorder have made contributions to our understanding, as in the work of Bruce Link and his colleagues. When consilient theories are developed, there will still be a need for approaches that are only one- or two-dimensional.

A second idea may be just as important, that of the devil's advocate. Biopsychiatry, the dominant force in the field, like all disciplines, accentuates the positive. Labeling theory can be considered to be a countertheory, critical of the weakest points in the dominant theory, and focusing on issues that it neglects. The two approaches can complement and correct each other, while we are awaiting Mr. Inbetween.

The original theory of mental illness presented in this book had its high-water mark in the 1970s, if perhaps only as a countertheory. During that decade labeling was taken seriously in sociology and, to a lesser extent, in anthropology, criminology, psychology, psychiatry, and social work. Its status began to wane in the next decade, and by the beginning of the 1990s it had been all but dismissed by the mainstream disciplines. As we shall see in Chapter 1, there are still proponents of the theory. But the majority of scholars and practitioners have moved on to other interests.

There are two main reasons for the loss of interest. The most important is what is called popularly "the tranquilizer revolution," and the accompanying rise of biological psychiatry. Beginning in the 1980s and reaching its peak in the mid-90s, most social scientists and practitioners formed the impression that the problem of mental illness had been solved, at least in principle. The public was persuaded by claims that the causes and treatment of mental illness had been shown to be biological. It was thought, and still is by many, that genetic causes of mental illness had been or would shortly would be found, and that psychoactive drugs could cure or at least safely control the symptoms of metal illness.

The first part of Chapter 1 will be devoted to exploring these claims. It seems now that although biological psychiatry has made advances, in the main its claims have still not been sufficiently substantiated. These matters are too complex to deal with briefly, so they will be raised in the next chapter.

A second reason for the declining interest in the theory was various critiques proposing that since labeling theory was not substantiated by empirical studies, it should be abandoned. The most important of these critiques were those by Gove (1980; 1982). As with biological psychiatry, it now appears that the critiques of the labeling theory of mental illness were overstated. In Chapter 1, I will respond to Gove's critique.

The earlier editions of this book were based on studies conducted during the period 1960–1982. Since that time, there have been many extraordinary changes in the field of mental illness: the introduction of psychoactive drugs on a massive scale; the discovery of the neurotransmitters; the hope of finding genetic causes of mental illness; the proliferation and development of psychological therapies; changes in the mental health laws governing commitment and treatment; and finally, an increase in the number and scope of social scientific studies of mental illness. (For a description of the effect of the first edition of this book on mental health laws, see the Appendix.) This edition updates the earlier ones, bringing these changes and their aftereffects into its purview. In addition to these changes in the field since 1984, there have also been changes in my own point of view since the time of the first edition. First, the changes related to my work on catharsis of emotions, as reflected in the book on this topic (1979). Second, my studies of the emotions of pride and shame (Scheff 1990; 1994; 1997; Scheff and Retzinger 1991), and the link between these emotions and the state of the social bond. Third, my interest in connecting the world of everyday life to the larger institutions in a society has directed my attention to dialogue as data (Scheff 1990; 1997). Finally, mostly as a result of my dialogue studies, I now think, like Wilson (1998), that it is imperative to integrate the separate disciplines that deal with human behavior.

These changes in point of view have had three main effects on this edition. First, they have led me to more strongly emphasize that the original labeling theory of mental illness, as presented in Chapters 3–5, is only one of many partial points of view. Each of these points of view is useful, but in the long run, it will be necessary to integrate the differing standpoints, especially the psychological, sociological, and biological approaches.

The second change involves increased emphasis on emotions and social bonds. The original theory was predominantly cognitive and behavioral. In this edition, emotions and relationships are introduced, with a special emphasis on the emotion of shame as a key component in stigma and in the generation of the societal reaction to deviance. I now emphasize the role of pride/shame as Durkheim's "social emotion," and the interplay of these emotions with social bonds. Since emotions and bonds are biological, psychological, and social, increasing emphasis on *the emotional/relational world,* largely invisible in Western civilization, may offer a bridge between the disciplines. The original labeling theory was blind to the emotional/relational world; it dealt only with extremes of societal labeling and denial. In this edition, I extend the theory to include more subtle forms of interaction.

Two of the new chapters (8 and 9) illustrate the emotional/relational world by applying labeling theory to the social interaction between therapist and patient. Chapter 8 involves a psychotherapy session between an anorexic woman, "Rhoda," and her therapist. The patient reports discourse in her family, especially dialogues between herself and her mother. These dialogues suggest that labeling of the patient occurred first in the family, before any formal labeling took place. This chapter points toward a modification and extension of the original theory.

Chapter 9 concerns the first meeting between an outpatient, "Martha," and a psychiatrist. It turns into a sparring match between the patient, who want to convey her emotional/relational world, and the psychiatrist, who wants to ascertain the facts. This interview exactly reverses the situation between therapist and client from that of the session in Chapter 8. In the latter session, it is the therapist who seeks to interest the client in her emotional/relational world. In the session in Chapter 9, it is the patient who tries to interest the psychiatrist in her (the patient's) emotional world. Because of her skill and patience, "Rhoda's" therapist is successful; she introduces her patient to the world of emotions. Martha's therapist, however, remains oblivious.

With respect to the original theory of labeling, after due consideration, I decided to revise mainly by addition rather than by making large changes in the original text (Chapters 3–5). A new Chapter 1 takes up the issues raised above about the perspective of biological psychiatry, on the one hand, and critiques of labeling theory, on the other. Because I was unable to find a very concise statement of the theory of social control, I wrote a new chapter for the second edition (Chapter 2), stating the main elements of social control and relating them to deviance and to mental illness.

I have resisted the temptation to make large changes in the text outlining the theory that was published in 1966 because it may still be useful in its original form. Since the discovery of the role of the neurotransmitters, and the impetus to genetic research provided by DNA, researchers who investigate schizophrenia and the other major mental illnesses believe that they are now asking the right questions, and that knowledge of the causes and cures of the major mental illnesses will be uncovered within their own lifetimes. This research, which grew out of the use of psychoactive drugs, has also convinced many psychiatrists that these drugs not only are important in the treatment of mental illness but also hold the key to the understanding and conquest of these problems. These are heady times for biological theories of mental disorder.

Although their hypotheses are plausible, they are still, at this writing, unproven. To date, no clearly demonstrable linkage between neurotransmission or genetics has been found for any major mental illness. The idea that the mentally ill suffer from deficient neurotransmission or genes is only a theory. Furthermore, even if the connection were made, most of the basic issues involving the social control of mental illness would remain. Since the connection is still hypothetical, it is premature to discard labeling theory.

The same reasoning applies to what has been popularly called the "tranquilizer revolution." As will be discussed in Chapter 1, even the most useful of the psychoactive drugs do not cure mental illness—they alleviate the symptoms. And again, even if a drug treatment were found that could cure mental illness, the fundamental issues of social control would remain. When the painkilling properties of morphine were discovered, physicians called it "God's own medicine," because they thought it was a cure. It took many years to realize that it was only a painkiller. There may be a parallel to be drawn between the discovery of morphine and that of psychoactive drugs. It has been less than fifty years since the large-scale use of tranquilizers began. It may still be too early to evaluate their overall effects.

I am not arguing that the neurotransmitter hypothesis is incorrect, or that drugs are worthless; I am only suggesting that it is much too early to discard labeling theory, despite the significant gains that have been made. Some balance is required in evaluating the competing claims of both the somatic and the social theorists. In its heyday, there was a tendency in sociology to overstate the claims of labeling theory. To avoid overstatement, in the 1984 edition I made two changes in the original text. First, I relinquished the "single most important" phrase in Proposition 9, stating instead that labeling is among the most important causes. The issue of the order of importance of the various causes is empirical anyway and should not have been reduced to a theoretical claim.

The second change involves qualifying the contrast between the two poles of the societal reaction. Originally, I called the reaction to deviance that was opposite to labeling "denial"; in this edition I have changed it to "normalization." In fact, denial is only one of many differing ways of reacting to deviance, such as rationalization, ignoring, and temporizing.

In the context of mental disorder it is important to note that treatment is not necessarily a labeling reaction. Labeling, in the sense I use it, always involves stigmatization; there is an emotional response as well as special label. Any form of response that does not stigmatize, such as skillful and humane psychotherapy and hospitalization, may also be a form of normalization. In some ways, the term *labeling* itself is perhaps unfortunate, since it has become fashionable to apply it to mere classification. What is needed is a more forceful term, one that would connote both labeling and stigmatization, so that a distinction could be made between reintegrative and rejecting classification, as in Braithwaite's (1989) approach to crime control.

It may help give perspective if I locate the labeling theory outlined in this book with respect to other "anti-psychiatry" approaches, as they have been called. Like the viewpoints of Goffman (1959), Laing (1967), and Szasz (1961), the theory in this book offers an alternative to the conventional psychiatric perspective. The basic difference from the other anti-psychiatry approaches is that I offer an actual *theory* of mental illness. That is, I propose a possible social scientific solution to the problem of defining and treating mental illness. The theory is made up of concepts that are at least partially defined, explicit causal hypotheses, and applications to real events. This theory is therefore testable, as Gove and others were able to show in the early critiques of the theory.

Although Goffman's approach is sociologically sophisticated, it does not contain a theory of mental illness. He defines his terms only conceptually, with little attention to the problem of goodness of fit to instances. Laing's approach is psychologically sophisticated, but involved even less conceptual development. Szasz, finally, uses no concepts; his approach is stated entirely in vernacular words. This approach makes it easy for anyone to understand, even laypersons. But it is much too narrow and simplified to use for analyzing and understanding actual cases, each of which is apt to be quite complex, like most human conduct.

Szasz makes the case that the medical model is not appropriate for most cases of what is designated to be mental illness and therefore that the term *mental illness* itself is inappropriate. I agree. But in order to make my argument understandable, I have resorted to that inappropriate terminology, only because it is coin of the realm. In this book, it should be understood that every time I use the term *mental illness* it should be seen as encased in quotation marks. My own terminology involves a sociological concept, as explained in Chapter 3, "residual deviance."

Szasz's reliance on vernacular words reduces his theory almost to caricature. For example, the terminology that Szasz suggests as an alternative to "psychiatric symptoms" is "problems in living." If adapted, this usage might help to destigmatize the sufferers. But the phrase is much too broad, since it encompasses a vast realm of problems. Unrequited love, overextension of one's credit, and the incapacities of old age are certainly all commonly encountered problems of living, but they are not the particular types of problems that are designated as mental illness. If Szasz had used the terminology "residual problems of living" (problems that don't have conventional names), he would have come close to my solution of the problem. In any case, a social theory requires statements of explicit hypotheses, all of which are couched in terms of conceptual and operational definitions. The labeling theory provides these, the other antipsychiatric formulations do not.

It is my hope that this edition will provide a clear statement of a sociological approach to mental disorder, and at least some small steps toward integrating it with other approaches to the understanding and treatment of mental disorder.

I

INTRODUCTION

1

Biological Psychiatry and Labeling Theory[1]

Although the last five decades have seen a vast number of studies of functional mental disorder, there is as yet no substantial, verified body of knowledge in this area, comparable, say, to medical knowledge of infectious diseases. At this writing, there is no rigorous and explicit knowledge of the cause, cure, or even a coherent classification of the symptoms of functional mental disorders (such as schizophrenia, depression, or anxiety disorders). Such knowledge as there is, is clinical and intuitive. Clinical knowledge in psychiatry and the other mental health therapies is large and impressive, but so far has not been formulated in a way that would be subject to verification by scientific methods.

During these five decades, most research on mental illness has sought to establish three main contentions:

Etiology (causation)	1.	The causes of mental illness are mainly biological.
Classification	2.	Types of mental illness can be coherently classified (DMS-IV).
Treatment	3.	Mental illness can be treated effectively and safely with psychoactive drugs.

My argument about these claims will be based on a highly selective review of the relevant literature. My emphasis, for the most part, is on those

3

studies that raise questions about the validity of the biopsychiatric approach. My review is probably as unrealistically negative as the biopsychiatric literature is unrealistically positive. A balanced review is yet to be made (for a recent attempt, see Chapter 3 of Mechanic 1999).

Many people have the impression that all three of the biopsychiatric goals have been reached. Articles by journalists usually assume as much. Indeed, most of the articles published in psychiatric journals at least imply that these three goals are already established or that they will be established shortly. They are taken for granted. Certainly in psychiatric practice it is now a truism that most cases of mental illness should be treated with psychoactive drugs. Indeed, many psychiatrists argue that it is unethical not to. Their effectiveness and safety is assumed not only by the majority of psychiatrists, but also by health maintenance organizations, which in insuring medical care, have come to have an enormous say in the practice of psychiatry. Needless to say, advertising by drug companies continuously brings these alleged truths before the public.

But these assumptions still have not been proven. The true picture is much more complex. In a recent editorial in the *American Journal of Psychiatry,* a biological psychiatrist (Tucker 1998) complained about the three goals. He argues that the system of classification developed in psychiatry (DMS-IV) does not actually fit many patients, and that it has only succeeded in distracting attention from the patient as a whole. His main objection, however, is that the syndromes outlined in DMS-IV are free-standing descriptions of symptoms. Unlike diagnoses of diseases in the rest of medicine, psychiatric diagnoses still have no proven link to causes and cures. As Tucker says, making a point about both classification and causation: "All of this apparent precision [in DMS-IV] overlooks the fact that as yet, we have no identified etiological [causal] agents for psychiatric disorders" (p. 159). This particular sentence exactly explodes the biopsychiatric bubble (see also Valenstein 1998).

This article is especially noteworthy because it appears in the flagship journal of the American Psychiatric Association, the main psychiatric association in the United States, the home country of biological psychiatry. The most widely read of all psychiatric journals, until 1998 it relentlessly promoted the threefold objectives of biological psychiatry. This direction now seems to have slightly shifted, however, suggesting that the dominance of biological psychiatry may be coming to an end.

A second article challenging the position of biological psychiatry was published in the same journal soon after the Tucker article, reviewing studies that support interpersonal causation in the origins and outcome of mental illness (Lewis 1998). Lewis proposes ten central premises of the interpersonal school of psychiatry, and reviews studies that show the effectiveness of secure adult relationships in undoing the adult consequences of destructive childhood experiences, and the role of well-functioning marriages in decreasing depression. The appearance of the editorial and the special article in the *AJP* that challenge fundamental tenets of biological psychiatry may signal the beginning of the end of its dominance.

Even during the years of biological dominance, there has been a steady stream of studies that raise crucial questions about each of the three major strands. The status of claims of biological causation and systematic classification have always been ambiguous. Obviously there have been significant advances in knowledge about the interaction of biological and nonbiological factors in mental illness. A representative study of rates of occurrence of schizophrenia in Finnish twins can serve as an example (Tienari and Wynne 1994). Tienari and Wynne found that the rate of schizophrenia in the "adopted-out" twin born to a schizophrenic mother was manyfold greater than in the population at large, suggesting a genetic factor. But on the other hand, even though the rates were high, still most of the adopted twins with a schizophrenic mother were not diagnosed as schizophrenic, suggesting a nongenetic origin.

To confirm a genetic cause, even for only one part of those diagnosed as schizophrenic, the deficit gene would have to be isolated. Although studies of DNA report promising areas of exploration, this step has yet to occur. Like the claim earlier in the century that psychoanalysis was on the threshold of a breakthrough, the claim of genetic causation seems premature (Grob 1998).

The classifications of psychiatric disorders that have been organized into the succeeding DSM versions appear to be little more than attempts to confirm current psychiatric practices, rather than empirical studies. Empirical studies usually show broad discrepancies between diagnostic categories and patient symptoms. An example is the study of symptom clusters by Strauss (1979), a widely respected research psychiatrist. He compared the actual cluster of symptoms that each of 217 first-admission patients displayed with the diagnostic syndromes. He concluded that the clusters of "the vast majority [of the patients] fall between syndromes." That is to say, the symptoms of the large majority of actual patients do not cohere the way the DSM organizes them, suggesting that, in this fundamental respect, the problems that psychiatrists treat do not seem to fit into the medical model of disease (also see Mirowsky 1990).

Researchers from social work have published two books suggesting that the DSM classifications are determined much more by the politics of psychiatry than by evidence (Kirk and Kutchins 1992; Kutchins and Kirk 1997). In the first book (1992) they show that evidence that would confirm the DSM classifications is vanishingly small.

The strongest strand of the biological revolution in psychiatry has always been treatment with psychoactive drugs. In the early years of their use, these drugs were seen as ways of controlling and dispelling the symptoms of mental illness, if not as absolute cures. Especially when compared to psychological and social measures, drugs were seen as being cheap, quick, safe, and effective. There is still no question about how quick, cheap, and easy to administer the drugs are. But in the last twenty years evidence that contradicts the effectiveness and safety of psychoactive drugs has been becoming available. There are also indications that these drugs may be administered to manage or control certain categories of patients, rather than to help them.

EFFECTIVENESS OF PSYCHOACTIVE DRUGS

There are a vast number of systematic studies that seem at first glance to testify to the effectiveness of psychoactive drugs. These are almost all what is called randomized clinical trials (RCTs), carried out using the standard design for scientific experiments. A group of patients with similar diagnoses are divided randomly into two subgroups. One subgroup, the treatment group, receives the drug, the other, the control group, gets an inert substance disguised as a medication, a "placebo." The design requires that the administration of the substances be "blind," that is, neither the patients nor the doctors know which are the drugs and which placebos. If the subgroups are set up at random, and if the participants are "blind," then any change in the treatment group larger than the control group can be confidently ascribed to the effects of the drug.

The usually positive results of these studies are thought to demonstrate two points: (1) that psychoactive drugs are more effective than the placebos used in the control groups, and (2) that their effectiveness is due to the correction of biological deficits in the patients. However it is important to note that even if these results are accepted at face value, the average difference in effect between the drug and the placebo group in the typical study is not large and is often short-lived, as shown in studies over time. Typically, in repeat studies done from four to eight months after the initial one, the average advantage of the treatment group over the control group has decreased or even disappeared. Since we are dealing with averages among many patients, this is not to say that there aren't strong positive and negative, and even no effects on individual patients. To summarize: even accepting the validity of the RCTs, most psychoactive drugs are only slightly and briefly more effective than placebos. The decreasing effectiveness over time is suggestive of a placebo effect.

In recent years many studies have challenged the standard interpretation of the RCT studies, that psychoactive drugs, in themselves, are more effective than inert substances, and that their effectiveness is due to the correction of biological deficiencies. It now appears that most RCTs are not truly blind, because most of the participants can make accurate guesses as to whether the patient is receiving a psychoactive drug. Shapiro and Shapiro (1997, Table 9.1) reviewed 27 studies that asked doctors, patients, and "raters" (outside observers) to guess who was receiving the drug.

On average, 93% of the doctors, 73% of the patients, and 67% of the raters could accurately guess the active agent. Doctors, patients, and raters can use physical effects, taste, color, texture, and dissolvability to guess. Especially for the patient, the physical effects on the body often reveal the active drugs, since many of them are powerful stimulants, sedatives, or emotion blockers. The drug companies who conduct most of the RCTs seldom try to make a close match between the drug and the placebo, because they think it is not sufficiently important to warrant investing in the complex task of precise matching. In a scholarly review of this issue, Healy (1997) is also critical of the use of RCTs in evaluating the effects of antidepressants.

In my opinion, even a careful attempt at precise matching would face an insoluble dilemma. If the placebo were precisely enough matched to the medication, then its own effects on the patient would make the results of the experiment ambiguous. I think that experimental designs that necessitate blind administration of medicine and placebo are inappropriate for human beings. Case studies are more appropriate. Although they also involve reliability problems, they are nearer to the surface. The RCTs hide validity and reliability problems behind the mask of hard science. For a proposal to apply the case study method to the problem of evaluating drug effects, see Jacobs and Cohen (1999).

If the great majority of the participants are not truly blind, then the validity of the entire method of research is thrown into question. The purpose of the RCT design is to rule out all explanations other than the biological effect on the patient. If most of the patients and doctors in the studies know which medications are active, the possibility arises that some or even most of the effects are psychological and/or social.

PLACEBO REACTIONS

This possibility is known as "the placebo effect." It has been documented that all substances prescribed by a physician, even if they are inert, can have powerful effects on the patient (Fisher and Greenberg 1997; Harrington 1997; Shapiro and Shapiro 1997). The processes that give rise to this effect are not well understood. It is believed, however, that the social psychology of hope, both in the doctor and in the patient, plays an important role.

Even in physical illness, the loss of hope can lead to deterioration of health independently of the disease process. For example, one study of 2,400 middle-aged men (Everson, Goldberg, and Kaplan 1996) found that hopelessness was the best predictor of death from heart disease and cancer. Six years after the initial interview, the 11% of the men with the highest level of hopelessness had died at three times the rate of the men who were hopeful. Hopelessness was the best predictor of death or illness even in those men who had no prior history of heart disease or cancer.

In mental illness, the effect of hope is probably still greater. Anything that can increase the patient's hopefulness can be potent medicine. In understanding the effects of psychoactive drugs on doctors and patients, it is important to remember that before "the tranquilizer revolution," many psychiatrists believed that there was nothing they could do to help their patients, especially their psychotic patients. Perhaps the chief effect of these drugs, particularly the anti-psychotic ones, has been on the psychiatrists, restoring their confidence in their own competence, and therefore their hope for the patients. The doctor's hope, quickly sensed by their patients, could increase the patient's own hope, and improve the relationship between doctor and patient, and therefore the whole social psychology of treatment of mental illness.

Of course many, many patients are themselves convinced that they have been helped by psychoactive drugs; they feel that the drugs they were given were instrumental in controlling their psychosis, depression, or anxiety. What is the harm to them if the help they got, in most cases, was entirely due to the placebo effect? This issue brings up the question of side effects of psychoactive drugs.

ARE PSYCHOACTIVE DRUGS SAFE?

Just as placebo effects accompany all substances prescribed by physicians, so also do side effects. It has been known for many years that some of the widely used anti-psychotic drugs (neuroleptics), such as Thorazine, cause neurological damage, even in small doses, if they are administered regularly (Cohen 1997). It is possible that all psychoactive drugs, including the mildest tranquilizers, have potent side effects. The side effects, unlike drug effectiveness, have not received enough direct research attention. Since the actions of most psychoactive drugs are complex and not understood, patients receiving them are being experimented on.

There are now many studies that demonstrate adverse effects of psychoactive drugs in a sizable minority of patients. Tardive dyskinesia is caused by Thorazine and other similar neuroleptics. If administered for as little as three months, even in low dosages, these medications will sooner or later cause severe neurological damage, tardive dyskinesia. In this syndrome, the patient loses control over his body, leading to involuntary spasms and tics that impair motor functions. Surprisingly, although this side effect is widely known, and many new neuroleptics have been introduced that are supposed to be less likely to cause it, Thorazine and the other offending drugs are still used widely (Cohen 1997).

Antidepressants have also been shown to have adverse side effects. One study (summarized by Ayd 1998) showed that these drugs led to profound apathy and indifference in 11% of the patients who receive the drugs. A second study (Settle 1998) reported that 20% of 207 consecutive admissions to a psychiatric hospital had psychoses caused by withdrawal from antidepressants. Surely in physical medicine any treatment that had such severe and frequent side effects would be peremptorily suspended from use. It is no longer clear that the benefits of psychoactive drugs outweigh the costs, even though a majority of psychiatrists, and all drug companies and HMOs, have persuaded themselves that this is the case.

In my own observations of persons who take psychoactive drugs, the reactions have been variable. In mental hospitals, by the middle of the eighties, virtually all of the patients were being given psychoactive drugs. Most of the patients were receiving at least two different drugs, some as many as five. Most of the patients I interviewed complained about adverse effects, hinting that they discarded the drugs. Some showed me how they were able to evade the drugs even if they were given them by nurses, by "mouthing" the drugs so that they could later dispose of them.

Some of my outpatient subjects were ambivalent about their drugs. Two of them had a quite similar reaction to lithium carbonate, a mineral still widely used to control mood swings in bipolar (manic-depressive) illness. Both reported that the mineral brought considerable relief from their mood swings, but also interfered with their mental and creative capacities. Both elected to discontinue.

On the other hand, a few of the hospital patients, and a majority of the people I knew as outpatients, told me that they were undoubtedly helped by their drugs, often spectacularly. In questioning them closely about drug effects, I usually found that these subjects were convinced to the point that they were impatient with my detailed questions. Some reminded me of persons who had had a religious conversion. They sang the praises of their drugs, and were not cooperative in responding to questions.

The psychiatrist Aaron Lazare (1989) found that many patients in the outpatient clinic he directed requested tranquilizers, even in cases when the psychiatrist thought other treatments were indicated. In response, Lazare developed a protocol he called "the negotiated approach to outpatient treatment," and trained his staff to use it. First the psychiatrist elicits a request from the patient, with a choice of 14 categories: advice, confession, succorance, ventilation, and so on. If the patient requested drugs, the psychiatrists were taught to give the patients brief demonstrations of alternative treatments, such as psychotherapy. Using this method, Lazare's clinic managed to reduce the number of patients on drugs to a level far lower than the average.

There is one further problem connected with the biological approach: the way it is used with vulnerable populations. It seems likely that it is frequently being used to control or manage children, confined aged persons, and women, rather than to help them. It is clear that the drug Ritalin is being used widely to control children whom teachers find difficult to manage (Breggin 1998; Diller 1998; DeGrandpre 1999; Walker 1998). Even a physician who prescribes their use admits that they are vastly overused (Diller 1998). Although not condemning the cautious use of Ritalin, Diller, like Breggin, DeGrandpre, and Walker, proposes that there is an epidemic of indiscriminate use for problems that are social or psychological rather than biological.

There is also scattered evidence that psychoactive drugs are administered indiscriminately to a majority of the elderly who are confined in convalescent and board and care homes: "[N]euroleptic medications are used in 39% to 51% of elderly institutionalized patients" (Lancetot et al. 1998). These figures refer only to anti-psychotic drugs. If antidepressants and other tranquilizers were included, the figures would be much higher. It may be that psychoactive drugs are being used as chemical straitjackets for a large majority of the confined elderly.

A sizable number of books and articles have protested the way in which psychiatric diagnosis and treatment systematically discriminates against women (for reviews, see Brown 1994; Lerman 1996; Tavris 1992). It would appear that what would likely be called symptoms of mental illness if they occur in women are apt to be ignored when they occur in men. Since the vast majority of psychiatrists, until quite recently, have been men, feminist commentators argue that male psychiatrists have usually discriminated against women in their diagnoses and treatment. They also argue that the DSM classification series has discriminated against women. For example, sexual behavior that would probably be ignored in men has been classed as psychopathy or hypersexuality in women:

[T]he concern over female autonomy that was implicit in the category of hypersexuality helps explain why psychiatrists considered failure to engage in heterosexual courtship—whether simple lack of interest or overtly lesbian behavior—just as psychopathic as a woman's too vigorous exercise of her seductive powers. (Lunbeck 1994, p. 522)

Although Lunbeck's comment concerns diagnostic practices earlier in this century at the Boston Psychopathic Hospital, evidence provided by Brown, Lerman, and Tavris suggest that it is still relevant to current practices.

CHALLENGING THE RULE OF BIOPSYCHIATRY

Biopsychiatry so dominates the whole field of mental illness that it is difficult to view the field from a different perspective. It is not easy to locate descriptions of practice that do not assume the three central principles of classification, causation, and treatment described above. To give an alternative view, I call upon a report by a psychiatrist who substituted for a vacationing regular at a managed care mental health clinic. This psychiatrist has asked that he not be identified for fear of retaliation:

> The clinic was privately run, but it had the state contract to provide the local community mental health. I chose not to speak openly about my views, but to lay low and keep quiet. . . . I did manage to lower the dose or discontinue the medications on most of the patients I saw. I was also able to get the court-ordered treatment rescinded on one patient, so all in all I was able to do some good . . .
>
> Here's what I learned: The whole mental health system seems to be relying almost exclusively on medications. If a patient requests medications, he is given it freely. If he requests any kind of counseling or therapy, he has to present his request before a review panel that will in most cases deny the request. When a patient was not doing well, everyone looked to me immediately to "adjust his medications." If the patient was already adequately medicated, then the assumption was that the patient must not be "compliant." No one ever seemed to consider the possibility that the medicines may not work, even if taken. Nearly every patient I saw was on multiple medications.
>
> The majority of patients on Lithium and Depakote were not being adequately monitored with the required blood tests (I diagnosed 4 cases of lithium-induced renal impairment that should have been detected long before). Tardive Dyskinesia was very prevalent but frequently undiagnosed or misdiagnosed. Even in diagnosed TD, the offending agent was not discontinued, except in a few cases. Most patients had no idea what medicines they were taking or why. They take the medicine because everyone wants them to, or in some cases because their continued SSI, housing, and other benefits depended on it. The whole system is infantilizing. Those people who take well to being infantilized, thrived in it (i.e., they became fully infantile). Those who didn't were considered difficult.
>
> I was hailed by the clinic staff and by many patients as a good psychiatrist, mostly because I was the first psychiatrist they had seen who bothered to talk with patients about their real problems. Apparently all other psychiatrists focus exclusively on medications and "symptoms." The progress note and psych eval forms they gave me to complete were fill-in-the-blank checklists that were exclusively symptom-oriented. If I wanted to note any sort of psychosocial issue (like the patient going through a divorce, etc.) I had to write it in the margin! I thought that pretty much said it all. I did a lot of scribbling in the margins in hopes that maybe someone would read it and be inspired to think of the person as a person, and not just as a set of symptoms.

Although this particular observation, based only on one clinic, may not be universally relevant, it is alarming enough to warrant at least some skepticism about biopsychiatry. It could well be the promised breakthrough, or it could also be a mere house of cards. It is too early to tell.

Given the lack of substantial knowledge of drug actions and effects, an attitude of patient study and observation would seem to be fitting for biopsychiatry at this time. All too often, however, mere hype is hidden by terminology. One example is the naming of the antidepressant drugs called SSRIs (systemic seratonin re-uptake inhibitors), like Prozac, Zoloft, and other similar drugs. A more modest procedure for naming would be to use the chemical class these drugs belong to, because the name SSRI prejudges the issue. Although there is substantial evidence that the amount of seratonin (a neurotransmitter) available to the brain is increased by these drugs, it is also known that they have many other complex effects, none of which are understood. It is conceivable that the positive drug effects are not due to seratonin, or at least not solely, but to one or more of the other effects (Thase and Kupfer 1996).

Given the overall picture of the lack of proof of genetic causation, the chaos of diagnosis, the small average efficacy and dangerous side effects of psychoactive drugs, and their abuse in vulnerable populations, why hasn't the biological approach been overthrown? The economics of drug use supplies part of the answer. It has been extremely profitable for drug companies to exaggerate the efficacy of psychoactive drugs, and to play down their brief effectiveness and destructive side effects. (For documentation of the drug companies' role in suppressing negative evidence, see Breggin 1991; Ross and Pam 1995; and Healy 1997.) It has also been profitable to the HMOs and to many of the psychiatrists who administer them.

The main alternative to drugs is psychotherapy, which is lengthy and extremely costly in comparison, and whose outcome is uncertain. HMOs much prefer paying $50 to $100 a month for medications than the at least $500 a month that four sessions of psychotherapy would cost. Similarly, the psychiatrist who dispenses drugs can schedule four patients an hour, rather than taking a whole hour for each psychotherapy patient. Being a psychotherapist rather than a pill prescriber also takes more skill, considerably more patience, and exerts more emotional wear and tear on the therapist. Identifying the emotional and relational tangles in a patient's life is not an easy task, requiring experience, patience, and self-confidence. Finally, psychoactive drugs give psychiatrists a competitive edge over other professionals who treat mental disorder, since only psychiatrists can prescribe them.

But independently of these incentives, there is also a powerful demand for drugs from patients and from their families. Drug treatment upholds the social and emotional status quo; individual and group psychotherapy can threaten it. Psychiatric approaches to the causes and treatment of mental disorder that focus on biology have been embraced wholeheartedly by the families of mental patients who support the National Alliance for the Mentally Ill (NAMI). To them, biopsychiatry seems to dismiss the possibility of familial causes and changes in the family system that might be required by social and psychological approaches. These families have bitterly rejected the idea that family relationships may be a cause of their relatives' mental disorder. Biological psychiatry, as they interpret it, seems to relieve them of dealing with shame and guilt, and indeed from any concern with their own behavior, emotions, and relationships. It leaves their family systems, no matter how slightly or extremely dysfunctional, inviolate.

THE EMOTIONAL/RELATIONAL WORLD

Like the dark side of the moon, the emotional/relational aspects of Western civilization are usually hidden from view. Western societies are highly oriented toward individualism and individual achievement (rather than toward groups and toward tradition, as in Asian and other traditional societies). Perhaps the clearest exposition of this doctrine was voiced by the American philosopher Emerson, in his philosophy of self-reliance. In one of his many paeans to the individual, he said: "When my genius calls, I have no father or mother, no brothers or sisters." This idea is exactly opposite to the ruling idea in traditional societies, that *nothing* comes before family, clan, or nation.

Unwittingly, Emerson's idea has become one of the main driving forces in Western societies. It prepares children for individual careers, enabling them to be social and geographically mobile so that they can avail themselves of opportunities for achievement, no matter at what personal and interpersonal cost. It has been one of the main forces leading to the suppression of emotions and the ignoring of personal relationships. One's feelings and the quality of one's personal relationships do not show up on résumés; they are dispensable. The relational world and its accompanying emotions have become virtually invisible in the Western middle-class world.

A classic example of the role of emotional/relational tangles in generating psychiatric symptoms was provided by a psychiatrist/sociologist team (Stanton and Schwartz 1954) in their study of patients in a mental hospital. Using case histories of symptom flare-ups, they demonstrated that each and every one was due to events in the patients' social environment. The feature common to all of their cases, they found, was covert disagreement among the staff about the patient. To unearth the actual cause of the flare-up took, in each case, patient and sometimes lengthy investigations. Even then, in the pre-tranquilizer era, there was considerable pressure to attribute the flare-up to the patient's illness, and to treat it with medication. The identification and correction of emotional/relational tangles is not a simple task, especially since it sometimes results in collisions with the egos of the participants and with the emotional/relational status quo in the organization or family.

Another example of social/emotional causation of symptom flare-up can be found in Retzinger's (1989) microanalysis of a psychiatric examination of a woman who had been previously diagnosed as schizophrenic. Taken from a widely used textbook on the initial psychiatric examination (Gill, Newman, and Redlich 1954), the flare-up of the patient's delusions is usually interpreted as an unpredictable outcome of the patient's illness. But Retzinger's close examination of the transcript tells a different story. She shows that the psychiatrist's (Fritz Redlich) manner initially was so warm and sympathetic that the patient responded to him in a patently sane and human way. The turning point comes when she notices that he has been glancing at the clock. Apparently threatened by being caught out by a supposedly insane patient, or perhaps worried about who is in control, Redlich's manner abruptly shifts. Without warning, he changes from a friend to a relentless diagnostician. He repeatedly probes and leads, trying to unearth the delusions reported in her record, to the point that she relapses into a delusional state. Retzinger calls Redlich's maneuver "reverting to technique," a subtle labeling and rejecting of the patient as a person. In this instance, the psychiatrist unwittingly shamed the patient into a delusional state.

The labeling that goes on in "Rhoda's" family (Chapter 10 in this book) is also subtle. In the dialogue between her and her mother that Rhoda reports in the therapy session, the mother never says directly that Rhoda is mentally ill, but she repeatedly implies that Rhoda is not a responsible person. Rhoda must understand this implication, because her emotional reactions are intense each time it occurs. The transcript on which this chapter is based is taken from another well-known text, an early microanalysis of a therapy session (Labov and Fanshel 1977).

Labov and Fanshel's reaction to their own analysis illustrates the elusiveness of the emotional/relational world in our civilization. At the end of the book, they note that if their analysis of the family dialogue reported by Rhoda is to be believed, then conflict is perpetual in that family: every line bristles with covert hostility, rejection, or withdrawal. But this idea troubles the authors, because it is also clear from the dialogue that Rhoda and her mother are both completely unaware of their emotional conflict; they recognize only physical violence (Rhoda is anorexic). Labov and Fanshel raise an astounding question: how could there be conflict if the participants are unaware of it? Opting to believe the participants rather than their own data, Labov and Fanshel disown their work, the emotional/relational world they themselves uncovered.

Biological approaches to mental illness support and help perpetuate the hiding of the emotional/relational world. This is a Durkheimian idea that I will discuss further later in this book. Preserving the inviolability, the sanctity of our avoidance of emotions and relationships can help explain the intensity of the societal reaction to mental illness. Biological psychiatry, in its crude popular form, is a collective representation that serves to maintain the emotional/relational scheme of things in our society.

GOVE'S CRITIQUE OF THE LABELING
THEORY OF MENTAL ILLNESS

In the seventies and early eighties, Walter Gove (1980; 1982) published several articles and two highly influential critiques of labeling theory. He proposed in these critiques that the evidence was so overwhelmingly negative that the theory should be abandoned. At least in mainstream studies in sociology and in related disciplines, his recommendation was nearly carried out. As a result of both the ascent of biological psychiatry and Gove's and other critiques, the great majority of researchers in social and medical science have virtually dismissed labeling theory as a fad of the sixties and seventies.

Since Gove's critique has been so influential, I will critique it in turn, in light of the evidence since the time that it was published. I cannot much criticize his review of the evidence at the time that he wrote. With some exceptions, the studies that sought to apply the theory found little or no support for it, just as he said. A clear and explicit general theory that is testable is a rarity in the social sciences. The survival of general theories like those of Marx and Freud are due, in least in part, to their vagueness. Quantitative researchers, whose forte is entirely given over to testing hypotheses, rather than generating them, fell upon labeling theory ravenously. They were encouraged also by the hubris of the original theorists, who overstated the importance of labeling.

By now, however, the situation has changed. In the last twenty years, a steady stream of studies has given a much more mixed picture. On the one hand, there are still plentiful studies that ignore labeling hypotheses, reject them on a conceptual basis, or, in some cases, once more find negative evidence. On the other hand, there are by this time a large number of studies that consistently report labeling effects. The best-organized series has been conducted by Bruce Link and his colleagues. For the period 1980 to 1990, Link and Cullen (1990) report eight of Link and his colleagues' own published studies, as well as those of others; they all show labeling effects in mental illness. More recent studies (Link et al. 1991; 1992; 1997) continue in the same vein.

To be sure, the continuing evidence for the labeling theory of mental illness is still sparse and mixed: a mixture of positive and negative findings. However, we now know that the evidence relevant to biological psychiatry is also mixed. As already indicated, there are now many studies that at least raise questions about the validity of genetic causation, the effectiveness and safety of psychoactive drugs, and the reliability of diagnostic classifications. There are also reasons to doubt the validity of the many studies of effectiveness and safety of drugs that were produced or sponsored by drug companies (for documentation of the exaggeration of positive evidence and suppression of negative evidence, see Breggin 1991; 1997).

Even acknowledging the initial spate of studies that failed to support the labeling theory of mental illness, Gove's recommendation that it be abandoned also arose out of the unfavorable comparison he made between labeling and psychiatric theory. Although his assessment of the evidence available at the time of his critique was mostly sound, his assessment of the validity of the psychiatric approach was not. He far overrated the coherence of diagnosis, the effectiveness and safety of drugs, and, indeed, the validity of the entire psychiatric approach. Given what we now know, Gove's view of psychiatry was naive. For this reason, it seems to me that the labeling theory of mental illness is still in the hunt. Of course, I am not suggesting that the other theories should be replaced by labeling theory, but only that mental illness, and indeed all human behavior, is still pretty much a mystery; competition between viable theories is still needed. In the next chapter I will discuss social systems and the relational/emotional world, steps toward a consilient (Wilson 1998) approach to the problem of mental illness.

NOTE

1.   My thanks to the efforts to remedy deficiencies in my knowledge of biopsychiatry by Peter Breggin, David Cohen, David Mechanic, Carlos Sluzki, and Douglas Smith.

2

Individual and Social Systems in Deviance

One frequently noted deficiency in psychiatric formulations is the failure to incorporate social processes into the dynamics of mental disorder. Although the importance of these processes is increasingly recognized by psychiatrists, the conceptual models used in formulating research questions are basically concerned with individual rather than social systems. Genetic, biochemical, and psychological investigations seek different causal agents but utilize similar models: dynamic systems that are located within the individual. In these investigations, social processes tend to be relegated to a subsidiary role, because the model focuses attention on individual differences rather than on the social system in which the individual is involved.

Even in the theories that are not organic in nature, the social system is relegated to a relatively minor place in the understanding of mental illness. This is true in psychoanalytic theory, the most influential of the non-organic theories, although Freud and his students frequently noted the importance of the social and cultural setting. In order to underscore the importance of the system properties of a theory, it is useful to compare psychoanalytic ideas, which are built around individual systems, with Marxist analysis, which is entirely social systemic and excludes completely any consideration of individual systems.

In psychoanalytic theory, the origins of neurosis are external to the individual. Freud's formulation was: "The Oedipus complex is the kernel of every neurosis." Fenichel, Freud's disciple and chief codifier of psychoanalytic

17

ideas, states: "The Oedipus complex is the normal climax of infantile sexual development as well as the basis of all neuroses" (1945, p. 108). For girls, the mirror image of the Oedipal complex is called the Electra complex. According to this theory, all children pass through a stage in which the parent of the opposite sex is chosen as a sexual object, causing intense hostility and rivalry toward the parent of the same sex. For children who go on to become normal adults, the Oedipal conflict is resolved: the child rejects the opposite-sex parent as a sexual object and identifies with the parent of the same sex. The rejection of the parent as a sexual object frees the child from later incestuous and therefore guilt-laden sexual impulses, and the identification with the same-sex parent begins the formation of the superego, which is the very basis for a normal adult psychic structure.

If, however, the opposite-sex parent is not rejected as a sex object and the same-sex parent not taken as a model, a fundamental fault is created in the psychic structure. In this case, the person grows into an adult who is never psychologically separated from his parents: Throughout his life, he is fighting and refighting the Oedipal conflict. All his relations with persons of the opposite sex are tinged with incestuous guilt, because his perceptions are based on his early childhood images in the family. Similarly, all his relations with same-sex persons are colored by the hostility and rivalry he felt for his parent of the same sex. According to this theory, the boy who goes through childhood without resolving the Oedipal conflict never establishes new relationships with women or men in later life but is imprisoned within the incestuous, and therefore psychologically untenable, relationship with his mother, and the hostile, rivalry-ridden relationship with his father.

Fenichel notes that the social situation in the child's family at the time of the Oedipal conflict is a key determinant of whether the conflict is resolved. The absence of one of the parents, or the weakness of one or the other as a model, as well as many other contingencies, is a potential cause of lack of resolution. It should be noted, however, that these external sources of defect are no longer involved in the neurotic system of behavior after the Oedipal stage passes (approximately from the ages of 3–7 years). If the Oedipal conflict is not resolved at this stage, the psychic flaw will continue throughout later life, more or less independently of later life experiences. It is true that psychoanalysts do speak of precipitating factors in adult life, but it is clear that these factors are of only subsidiary interest. The person in the throes of the Oedipal conflict is a defective adult, such that stresses that others could easily surmount might plunge him into a full-scale neurosis.

Thus the psychoanalytic model of neurosis is basically a system of behavior that is contained within the individual. The external situation in which the individual is involved is seen only as an almost limitless source of triggers for a fully developed neurotic conflict within the individual. Psychoanalytic theory, like most contemporary theories of mental illness, whether they are psychological or organic, locates the neurotic system within the individual. To be sure, psychoanalysts, like other psychological theorists, allow for external causation Fenichel (1945) states:

> The normal person has few "troops of occupation" remaining at the position "Oedipus complex," to use Freud's metaphor, the majority of his troops having marched on. However, under great duress they, too, may retreat, and thus a normal person may become neurotic. The person with a neurotic disposition has left nearly all his forces at the Oedipus complex; only a few have advanced, and at the slightest difficulty they have to go back and rejoin the main force at their first stand, the Oedipus complex. (p. 108)

Similar disclaimers can be found in virtually all the current theories of mental illness. Needless to say, in these theories, as in psychoanalytic theory, the direction and thrust of the perspective is found not in these exceptions and qualifications, but in systemic linkages that they posit, connecting key characteristics of individuals with their neurotic behavior. In psychoanalytic theory, the great conceptual development occurs in linking the origins of neurosis in the Oedipal stage through the mechanisms of psychosexual development to their end result, which is treated by the psychoanalyst theoreticians in a great wealth of detail: the formations of dreams, everyday slips and errors, and finally, in their manifold variety and complexity, neurotic symptoms.

Many of the critics of psychoanalytic theory have focused on just this feature as objectionable: the tracing of the most diverse kinds of human reactions back to the generic psychological substructure resulting from the Oedipal conflict. Freud's critics claim that the psychoanalytic model of man is too tight, narrow, rigid, and one-dimensional. The way in which psychoanalysts have sought to show how artistic creativity derives from psychosexual conflict is a case in point. Critics have also objected to Freud's key postulate of the "overdetermination" of symptoms. The literature of psychoanalysis abounds in instances showing how a symptom is not simply a consequence of a single cause but is merely one aspect of a veritable network of psychic phenomena. It is for this reason that psychoanalysts are usually adverse to the treatment of symptoms: their theory leads them to expect that if a symptom is removed, without changing the basic psychological structure, a new symptom will shortly appear in its place. But critics have objected that psychoanalytic theory seems to posit a type of predestination in which the neurotic is prisoner of his inexorable neurotic system.

From the point of view of the construction of a viable scientific theory, however, much of this criticism seems misplaced. It is just the "systemness" of psychoanalytic theory that makes it such a powerful intellectual weapon for the investigation of neurotic behavior. Starting from relatively few general postulates, it develops an enormous number of propositions about very concrete types of behavior. Such a theory is both powerful, in that it ramifies into many areas of behavior, and at least potentially refutable, so that with an adequate program of empirical research it could be qualified, transformed, or rejected.

Furthermore, the notion of the overdetermination of symptoms is very much in accord with recent developments in theory construction. In general systems theory, for example, the idea of overdetermination is closely related to the model of a self-maintaining system. The key feature of such a system is "negative feedback," that is, deviations from the system's steady state are detected and fed back into the system in such a way as to cause the system to return to its steady state. There is no reason to believe that such a system is found in only biological or electronic realms; psychoanalytic interpretations have suggested many ways in which psychological systems have this property. In the discussion in the following chapters, a system with self-maintaining properties composed of the deviant and those reacting to him will be delineated.

The objection to psychoanalytic theory that is made here is not that it posits neurotic behavior as part of a closed system, but that the system that it formulates is too narrow, in that it leaves out aspects of the social context that are vital for understanding mental disorder. The basic model upon which psychoanalysis is constructed is the disease model, in that it portrays neurotic behavior as unfolding relentlessly out of a defective psychological system that is entirely contained within the body. To bring the individual systemic character of psychoanalytic theory into high relief, it is instructive to contrast it with Marxian theory, which is social systemic.

Like Freud, Marx began his analysis with relatively few, but highly abstract postulates. Chief among these postulates is the dictum that in any society the mode of production determines the basic social forms, including the economic and political systems, the direction and pace of social change, and, ultimately, even man's consciousness. This point is made very clearly when Marx states that the mode of production is the substructure and all other forms mere superstructure in any society. Marx went on to construct from this basic premise a theory of history and of society in which the characteristics of individuals are more or less irrelevant.

In his analysis of then contemporary Europe, Marx posited the accumulation of capital as the process that determined social structure and social change. In primitive capitalism, the critical step was the accumulation of sufficient capital that a man's subsistence was not continually in jeopardy. The early capitalist could afford to bargain for the labor he hired rather than accept whatever the market offered. Society was transformed into two classes: those who were in a bargaining position (the capitalists) and those who were not (the workers). In the course of bargaining, the market rates for labor inevitably assumed the bottom limit, the cost of the worker's subsistence, and the capitalists, by the same logic, inevitably waxed rich at the worker's expense. For our purposes, the interesting feature of Marx's theory was the manner in which it disregarded the motivations of the individuals involved. For the capitalists, for example, it did not matter whether they were humanitarian or not for the development of the capitalist system. A capitalist, who, for humane reasons, refused to expropriate the workers, would himself be expropriated by other capitalists. Marx and his followers felt that they had evolved a theory that was independent of the psychology of individuals.

From these considerations, Marx (1906) stated the law of capital accumulation:

> But all methods for the production of surplus value are at the same time methods of accumulation: and every extension of accumulation becomes again a means for the development of those methods. It follows therefore that in proportion as capital accumulates, the lot of the laborer, be his payment high or low, must grow worse. The law, finally, that always equilibrates the relative surplus-population, or industrial reserve army, to the extent and energy of accumulation, this law rivets the laborer to capital more firmly than the wedges of Vulcan did Prometheus to the rock. It established an accumulation of misery, corresponding with accumulation of capital. Accumulation of wealth at one pole is, therefore, at the same time accumulation of misery, agony of toil, slavery, ignorance, brutality, and mental degradation, at the other pole. (pp. 708–709)

Marx (1906) notes the social and psychological effect of this process on the individual laborer:

> Within the capitalist system all methods for raising the social productiveness of labor are brought about at the cost of the individual laborer; all means for the development of production transform themselves into domination over, and exploitation of, the producers; they mutilate the laborer into a fragment of a man, degrade him to the level of an appendage of a machine, destroy every remnant or charm in his work and turn it into a hated toil; they estrange from him the intellectual potentialities of the labor process in the same proportion as science is incorporated in it as an independent power; they distort the conditions under which he works, subject him during the labor process to a despotism the more hateful for its meanness; they transform his life-time to a working time, and drag his wife and child beneath the wheels of the Juggernaut of capital. (p. 708)

Beginning with the dynamics of the economic system, Marx developed propositions that led finally to a prediction of psychological consequence for individuals. The statement concerning estrangement from the intellectual potentialities of labor, together with other similar statements, is one basis for current formulations about alienation, a psychological condition that is of great interest in current social science.

For the purposes of this discussion, the failures of Marxian theory are not as important as the general form it takes. The rise of effective industrial unions vitiated Marx's analysis near its premise, the irreversibility of the law of capital accumulation. The form of his theory, however, provides an example of a social systemic model that does not include any aspects of individual systems of behavior. The question raised by this comparison is this: can we formulate a theory that somehow integrates both the individual and social systems of behavior?

Several sociologists and psychiatrists developed an approach that gives more emphasis to social processes than does traditional psychiatric theory yet does not entirely neglect individual aspects. Lemert (1951), Erikson (1957), and Goffman (1959), among sociologists, and Szasz (1961) and Laing and Esterson (1964), among psychiatrists, have contributed notably to this approach. Lemert, particularly, by rejecting the more conventional concern with the origins of mental symptoms and stressing instead the potential importance of the societal reaction in stabilizing rule-breaking, focuses primarily on mechanisms of social control. The work of all these authors suggests research avenues that are analytically separable from questions of individual systems and point, therefore, to a theory that would incorporate social processes.

In his discussion of gamesmanship, Berne (1964) offers an analysis of alcoholism that is based on a social system model rather than on an individual system model of alcoholism:

> In game analysis there is no such thing as alcoholism or "an alcoholic," but there is a role called the Alcoholic in a certain type of game. If a biochemical or physiological abnormality is the prime mover in excessive drinking—and that is still open to some question—then its study belongs in the field of internal medicine. Game analysis is interested in something quite different—the kinds of social transactions that are related to such excesses. Hence the "Alcoholic."
>
> In its full flower this is a five-handed game, although the roles may be condensed so that it starts off and terminates as a two-handed one. The central role is that of the Alcoholic—the one who is "it"—played by White. The chief supporting role is that of Persecutor, typically played by a member of the opposite sex, usually the spouse. The third role is that of Rescuer, usually played by someone of the same sex, often the good family doctor who is interested in the patient and also in drinking problems. In the classical situation the doctor successfully rescues the alcoholic from his habit. After White has not taken a drink for six months they congratulate each other. The following day White is found in the gutter.
>
> The fourth role is that of the Patsy, or Dummy. In literature this is played by the delicatessen man who extends credit to White, gives him a sandwich on the cuff and perhaps a cup of coffee, without either persecuting him or trying to rescue him. In life this is more frequently played by White's mother, who gives him money and often sympathizes with him about the wife who does not understand him. In this aspect of the game, White is required to account in some plausible way for his need for money—by some project in which both pretend to believe, although they know what he is really going to spend most of the

money for. Sometimes the Patsy slides over into another role, which is a help-ful but not essential one: the Agitator, the "good guy" who offers supplies with-out even being asked for them: Come have a drink with me (and you will go downhill faster).

The ancillary professional in all drinking games is the bartender or liquor clerk. In the game "Alcoholic" he plays the fifth role, the Connection, the di-rect source of supply who also understands alcoholic talk, and who in a way is the most meaningful person in the life of any addict. The difference between the Connection and the other players is the difference between professionals and amateurs in any game: the professional knows when to stop. At a certain point a good bartender refuses to serve the Alcoholic, who is then left without any supplies unless he can locate a more indulgent Connection. (pp. 73–74)

Berne seems to be suggesting that the dynamics of alcoholism have less to do with the motivations and traits of the alcoholic than with the interactions between the occupants of the five interpersonal positions that he describes. According to his analysis, alcoholic behavior is understandable only as an integral part of an interpersonal system.

A critique of the use of the medical model in psychiatry that parallels many aspects of the present discussion has been made by learning theorists in psy-chology. A thorough and well-documented statement can be found in the introduction to *Case Studies in Behavior Modification* (Ullman and Krasner 1965). The psychological model that is proposed as an alternative to the medical model is based on the stimulus-response arc. The resultant processes of diagnosis and treatment have been described simply by Eysenck (1959): "Learning theory does not postulate any such 'unconscious cause,' but re-gards neurotic symptoms as simple learned habits; there is no neurosis under-lying the symptom, but merely the symptom itself. Get rid of the symptom and you have eliminated the neurosis" (61–75; quoted in Ullman and Kras-ner 1965). The approach to mental disorder proposed by these researchers appears to be superior to the medical model in three ways: First, it is behav-ioral and therefore allows for empirical research. Second, it is related to a systematic and explicitly stated body of propositions (i.e., learning theory). Finally, it is supported by a sizable body of empirical studies. It seems clear that this approach has made important contributions to psychiatric theory and practice and is likely to lead to fruitful work in the future.

At the same time, it should also be noted that "behavior modification," in practice, tends to be used as an individual system model of mental disorder. Conceptually, this is not necessarily the case. Ullmann and Krasner concep-tualize psychiatric symptoms as maladaptive behavior. They go on to say that the goal of treatment of maladaptive behavior should be to change the pa-tient's relationship to environmental stimuli. This formulation does not pre-judge the question of whether the relationship should be changed by chang-ing the patient or the environment. But in listing the techniques used in behavior modification, it is clear that the target for these techniques is the patient. Such techniques as "assertive responses, sexual responses, relaxation responses, conditioned avoidance responses, feeding responses, chemotherapy, expressive therapy, emotive imagery, *in vivo* presentation of disruptive stimuli, modeling, negative practice, self-disclosure, extinction, selective positive reinforcement, and stimulus deprivation and satiation" are the major techniques listed by Ullmann and Krasner. These techniques are oriented toward changing the patient's psychological system rather than the interpersonal or social system of which he is a member. Furthermore, it is not clear how it is possible for the therapist to effect changes through conditioning when in actual fact the technique utilized by the therapist constitutes only a small fraction of the total environmental stimulation to which the patient is exposed.

Like the medical model, "behavior modification" tends to isolate the symptom from the context in which it occurs. This occurs even in carefully formulated statements such as the following of Ullmann and Krasner (1965). In their statement, they are very careful to relate maladaptive behavior to the social context:

> Maladaptive behaviors are learned behaviors, and the development and maintenance of a maladaptive behavior is no different from the development and maintenance of any other behavior. There is no discontinuity between desirable and undesirable modes of adjustment or between "healthy" or "sick" behavior. The first major implication of this view is the question of how a behavior is to be identified as desirable or undesirable, adaptive or maladaptive. The general answer we propose is that because there are no disease entities involved in the majority of subjects displaying maladaptive behavior, the designation of a behavior as pathological or not is dependent upon the individual's society. (p. 20)

To this point, their formulation concerning "maladaptive behavior" exactly parallels the definition of deviant behavior presented here. They go on to further specify the meaning of maladaptive behavior in terms of roles and role reinforcement.

> Specifically, while there are no single behaviors that would be said to be adaptive in all cultures, there are in all cultures definite expectations or roles for functioning adults in terms of familial and social responsibility. Along with role enactments, there are a full range of expected potential reinforcements. The person whose behavior is maladaptive does not fully live up to the expectations for one in his role, does not respond to all the stimuli actually present, and does not obtain typical or maximum forms of reinforcement available to one of his status. . . . Maladaptive behavior is behavior that is considered inappropriate by those key people in a person's life who control reinforcers. (p. 20)

Restated in sociological terms, their formulation is that deviance is the violation of social norms and leads to negative social sanctions. Again, the parallel between the psychological and the sociological formulation is quite close.

This formulation of maladaptive behavior in terms of role expectations and reinforcement is potentially a powerful psychological tool, since it tends to bring in the mechanisms of social control and provides a strong link, therefore, between individual and social system models of behavior. To maintain this link, however, it is necessary to remember that the classification of behavior as maladaptive is made relative to the standards of some particular society and is not an absolute judgment. (The same reasoning is applicable, of course, to the concept of deviance.)

It appears to be very difficult to maintain a relativistic stance when the individual system models are used, particularly when the framework is transmitted to students. An instance of this difficulty is represented by the interpersonal psychiatry of Harry Stack Sullivan and his students. Although Sullivan sought to take psychiatric symptoms out of the patient by defining them as disorders of interpersonal relationships, his students put them back in by defining mental illness as a deficiency in the *capacity* for interpersonal relations. This individualization of social system concepts can be seen in the Ullmann and Krasner formulation, when they define one criterion of maladaptive behavior as not responding to "all the stimuli actually present." Since the response to stimuli of anyone in any role is highly selective, it would seem that the definition at this point had reverted to the absolute definition of deviance in terms of individual pathology. One function of a social system model of mental disorder is to provide a framework for research that facilitates an approach to mental disorder that is free of the questionable assumptions of inherent pathology in psychiatric symptoms.

Of the formulations of anthropologists, the one that most nearly parallels the model described here is the biocultural model of Anthony F. C. Wallace (1961). Giving somewhat more emphasis to organic sources of rule-breaking, Wallace posits that the initial cause of mental illness is physiological, but that the cultural "mazeways" (cognitive maps) profoundly shape the course of illness. In some detail, he notes how the "theories" of illness of the sick individual, his family and associates, and the "professionals" impinge on illness as a behavior system. The chief components of a "theory" of illness are to be:

1. The specific states (normalcy, upset, psychosis, in treatment, and innovative personality).
2. The transfer mechanisms that explain (to the satisfaction of the member of the society) how the sick person moves from one state to another.

3. The program of illness and recovery that is described by the whole system.

Wallace gives an extended analysis of one particular syndrome, the Eskimo *pibloktoq,* an acute excitement sometimes known as Arctic hysteria. According to his theory, *pibloktoq* has a physiological base in calcium deficiency (hypocalcemia) but is shaped by the culture-bound interpretations made by the sick persons and those who deal with him. Following Wallace's model, Fogelson (1965) presents a detailed analysis of *windigo,* a syndrome of compulsive cannibalism reported among Northern Algonkian-speaking Indians, which emphasizes culture-bound interpretations of rule-breaking behavior. The relationship between Wallace's model and the model developed here will be discussed later (Chapter 10).

The purpose of the present discussion is to lead to, in the next two chapters, a set of nine propositions that make up basic assumptions for a social system model of mental disorder. This set is largely derived from the work of Wallace and Fogelson, all but two of the propositions (Propositions 4 and 5) being suggested, with varying degrees of explicitness, in the cited references. By stating these propositions explicitly, this theory attempts to facilitate testing of basic assumptions, all of which are empirically unverified or only partly verified. By stating these assumptions in terms of standard sociological concepts, the relevance to studies of mental disorder of findings from diverse areas of social science, such as race relations and prestige suggestion, are shown.

This theory also delineates three problems that are crucial for a sociological theory of mental disorder: What are the conditions in a culture under which diverse kinds of rule-breaking become stable and uniform? To what extent, in different phases of careers of mental patients, are symptoms of mental illness the result of conforming behavior? Is there a general set of contingencies that lead to the definition of deviant behavior as a manifestation of mental illness? Finally, this discussion attempts to formulate special conceptual tools that are directly linked to sociological theory to deal with these problems. The social institution of insanity, residual rule-breaking, deviance, the social role of the mentally ill, and the bifurcation of the societal reaction into the alternative reactions of normalization and labeling are examples of such conceptual tools.

These conceptual tools are utilized to construct a theory of mental disorder in which psychiatric symptoms are considered to be labeled violations of social norms and stable "mental illness" is considered to be a social role. The validity of this theory depends upon verification of the nine propositions listed in future studies and should therefore be applied with caution and with appreciation for its limitations. One such limitation is that the theory attempts to account for a much narrower class of phenomena than is usually found under the rubric of mental disorder; the discussion that follows will be focused exclusively on stable or recurring mental disorder and does not explain the causes of single episodes. A second major limitation is that the theory probably distorts the phenomena under discussion. Just as the individual system models understress social processes, the model presented here probably exaggerates their importance. The social system model "holds constant" individual differences in order to articulate the relationship between society and mental disorder. Ultimately, a framework that encompassed both individual and social systems and distorted the contribution of neither would be desirable. Given the present state of formulations in this area, this framework may prove useful by providing an explicit contrast to the more conventional medical and psychological approaches and thus assist in the formulation of socially oriented studies of mental disorder.

It should be made clear at this point that the purpose of this theory is not to reject psychiatric and psychological formulations in their totality. It is obvious that such formulations have served and will continue to serve useful functions in theory and practice concerning mental illness. The author's purpose, rather, is to develop a model that will complement the individual system models by providing a complete and explicit contrast. Although the individual system models of mental disorder have led to gains in research and treatment, they have also systematically obscured some aspects of the problem. The social system model, like the psychological model, highlights some aspects of the problem and obscures others. It does, however, allow a fresh look at the field, since the problems it clarifies are apt to be those that are most obscure when viewed from the psychiatric or medical point of view.

The case for the use of limited analytic models was clearly stated by Max Weber (1949), for analysis that he called "one-sided":

> The justification of the one-sided analysis of cultural reality from specific "points of view" . . . emerges purely as a technical expedient from the fact that training in the observation of the effects of qualitatively similar categories of causes and the repeated utilization of the same scheme of concepts and hypotheses offers all the advantages of the division of labor. It is free of the charge of arbitrariness to the extent that it is successful in producing insights into interconnections which have been shown to be valuable in the causal explanation of concrete historical events. (p. 71; quoted by Mechanic 1963, p. 167)

It can be argued that in addition to the advantages of the division of scientific labor as suggested by Weber, there is yet another advantage to one-sided analysis. In the nature of scientific investigation, a central goal is the development of the "crucial experiment," a study whose results allow for the decisive comparison of two opposing theories, such that one is upheld and the other rejected. Implicit in the goal of the crucial experiment is the conception of science as an adversarial process in which scientific progress arises out of the confrontation of explicitly conflicting theories. In his formulation of the history of change in the natural sciences, Kuhn (1962) considers all scientific progress as the conflict between "competing paradigms" (i.e., opposing theories). Whitehead has stated this view very clearly: "A class of doctrines is not a disaster—it is an opportunity. . . . In formal logic, a contradiction is the signal of a defeat; but in the evolution of real knowledge it marks the first step in progress towards a victory" (pp. 266–267).

One road of progress in science is the intentional formulation of mutually incompatible models, each incomplete and each explicating only a portion of the area under investigation. The advance of science, as in the theory of adversarial procedures in law, rests on the dialectical process that occurs when incommensurate positions are placed in conflict. In the present discussion of mental illness, the social system model is proposed not as an end in itself but as the antithesis to the individual system model. By allowing for explicit consideration of these antithetical models, the way may be cleared for a synthesis, a model that has the advantages of both the individual and the social system models but the disadvantages of neither.

II

THEORY

3

Social Control as a System

Social scientists look at deviance in a somewhat different way from other members of the society. In order to understand deviance objectively (the sense in which I use this term will be defined shortly), they argue, one must first understand the more general phenomena of social control, the processes that generate conformity in human groups. This chapter introduces the theory of social control and shows how it applies to nondeviant areas such as clothing and appearance, language, facial expressions, feeling, and thought. Subsequent chapters demonstrate how this theory may be applied to the phenomenon of mental illness.

Rather than start the discussion of social control abstractly, I indicate some elements of social control in a concrete area, that of clothing and appearance. What determines the way people dress? In particular, why is there so much uniformity in dress within a given social group? We feel that we understand why soldiers wear uniforms, but why do corporation executives, sorority women, and college professors, for example? Perhaps one could explore his or her own choice of clothing. What determines one's style of dress or the choice of items in one's wardrobe? This may not be an easy question to answer. If that is the case, try reviewing the process that went into the choice of each particular garment. One may say, "I don't care what other people think, I dress to please myself." Even if it were true literally that one dresses only to please oneself, it is probably not true that the opinions of others have

31

no impact at all. Some person's dress expresses the message: "I don't care what you think." Dressing to express this message betrays a form of social influence, if only a negative one. One may extend the exploration of the influences on one's appearance by reviewing how the significant people in one's life view your appearance. Such an exploration should reveal a great deal, not only about oneself but also about the process of social control as it applies to oneself.

The social control of clothing has been evoked succinctly by Quentin Bell (1967):

> There is . . . a whole system of morality attached to clothes and more especially to fashion, a system different from and frequently at variance with that contained in our laws and our religion. To go to the theatre with five days' beard, to attend a ball in faultless evening dress . . . but with your braces outside, instead of within your white waistcoat, to scatter ink on your spats, to reverse your tie, these things are not incompatible with moral or theological teaching, the law takes no cognizance of such acts. Nevertheless such behavior will excite the strongest censure in "good society." . . . [I]t is not however sheer lunatic eccentricity such as the absence of trousers or a wig worn back to front which excites the strongest censure; far worse are those subtler forms of incorrect attire: the "wrong" tie, the "bad" hat, the "loud" skirt, the "cheap" scent, or the flamboyant checks of the overdressed vulgarian. Here the censure excited is almost exactly comparable to that occasioned by dishonorable conduct. (p. 18)

Although some of the terms are British, the sentiments apply equally well to American society. In this excerpt, Bell makes an important point: nonconformity to community standards concerning appropriate dress can excite a very strong negative response from others. Furthermore, Bell notes, the community standards concerning clothing are not legal standards or religious standards. They may have no formal status at all. They seem to be unwritten or even, in some cases, unstated rules. Yet in spite of their informal status, they would appear to exert great influence over dress and appearance. This issue will be discussed later under the topic of formal and informal norms.

Bell goes on to make a second important point about social control that concerns the relationship between individual and collective feelings with respect to dress:

> It is not simply the judgment of society which acts upon the individual. Our confusion when, having sat for two hours on the platform of a public meeting, we discover that we have been wearing odd socks, our still worse confusion when we find that our flies have been undone (even though nothing of any consequence has been revealed) has something of the quality of guilt. Indeed, I think it may frequently happen here, as in other moral situations, that the offender may be not simply the worst but in fact the only sufferer. A rebellious collar stud, a minute hole in a stocking may ruin an evening without ever being

observed by the company at large. . . . "A sense of being perfectly well dressed,"
a lady is reported as saying to Emerson, "gives a feeling of inward tranquillity
which religion is powerless to bestow." (p. 19)

Again, Bell makes an important point: The power of social control is not limited to the operation of actual censure but includes the operation of imagined censure. We all have suffered excruciating agonies of embarrassment
in situations where the negative response of others to our appearance was
mostly or even entirely in our imagination. Social control seldom operates
so that individuals are passive recipients of others' responses: each person
plays an active role both by imagining future responses of others and by defining present actions of others as responses to one's own behavior. Each individual's actions both create and are created by social control. I will return to
this idea shortly in the discussion of the part that self-control plays in social
control.

In light of this discussion, a preliminary answer now can be given to the
question concerning the uniformity in clothing that we see around us. Social
control plays an important part in generating uniformity of dress and appearance. Social control involves the rewarding of conformity to shared expectations and the punishment of nonconformity. Clothing that conforms to the
group standards of dress is rewarded with praise and admiration. If it does
not conform, it is likely to generate criticism or disapproval.

The theory of social control is the major interpretive model in social science. It is for this reason that social scientists see deviance as a type of nonconformity and seek to understand deviance in terms of the operation of
social control. This approach to deviance is distinctive to social science, separating it both from the view of laypersons, on the one hand, and from the
experts on deviance like psychiatrists and police, on the other.

The social science approach to deviance is distinctive in three major ways.
First, both laypersons and professionals who deal with deviants usually see
deviance as mostly an individual matter; that is, they take an individual perspective toward deviance. What was it in the character and background of
the deviant that caused him to become deviant? How can her deviance be
stopped? Social scientists do not rule out these questions. But their framework
is broader in that it deals both with the individual deviant and with societies'
response. The individual perspective and the social control perspective are
alternative ways of understanding deviance.

An example illustrates how the social control perspective is broader than
the individual perspective. At a conference on child development, there
was a discussion of the disruptive behavior of two "hyperactive" children in
a class of 30 fifth-graders. The participants were focusing on the possible
causes of the hyperactivity in the backgrounds of the children and the tactics
that the teacher might use in managing their hyperactivity, including referral

to a physician who might prescribe tranquilizing drugs. However, I had remembered that in initially describing the situation, the observer who had introduced the case had said that the teacher spoke in a monotone and was dull. I suggested that we might discuss a question alternative to the one on the table: what was wrong with the other 28 children that they also were not disruptive but tolerated dull teaching? Although not all of the participants accepted the idea, it did lead to a restructuring of the discussion to include more of the larger context in which "hyperactivity" was taking place.

There are two distinctive ways of conceptualizing the sources of behavior: in the person or in the situation. Why don't my children do their homework? Perhaps because they are lazy. This answer puts the source of behavior in the children and ignores the context. An alternative answer would be because the homework is too difficult or too easy: they are not motivated by the task or the teacher. This answer puts the source of behavior in the context and ignores the children. Needless to say, any thoughtful analysis should allow for an examination of both the individuals and the context. Often the individual perspective on the sources of behavior is a somewhat disguised aspect of the naive societal reaction: ignore the context, place the cause for deviance in negative traits inside the rule-breakers, and punish them. Dewey put the matter succinctly: "Give a dog a bad name and hang it."

There is a second major way in which the social science concept of deviance is distinctive. The concept of deviance itself is used in a dispassionate way, stripped of the opprobrium the word ordinarily carries. It means a violation of social norms that usually brings stigma and a strong negative reaction from others. Deviance is the violation of those rules that are felt to be worthy of high respect. Not all rule-breaking excites a negative reaction. In different times and places, the breaking of rules may be seen as innovative, creative, comical, or not worthy of notice. But when important emotionally weighted norms are broken, such as those upholding loyalty to one's country, strong feelings of outrage are usually mobilized. The violation of such norms is deviance in the sociological sense.

The sociologist, however, seeks to apply the term only in a relative sense: in a certain tribe, looking directly at the emperor's face is a deviant act—it causes outrage in the members of the tribe but not to the sociologist as an outsider. When the sociological concept of deviance is applied to one's own society, it requires an attitude of alienation, using the term as if it did not carry opprobrium to us, the users, but only to the other un-self-conscious members of the society. The first lesson in this discussion is that sociological analysis can be alienating. It requires that the analyst be stationed outside of his/her own society.

Alienation is the sense that elements of one's own life are meaningless. Churchgoers sometimes feel they are merely going through the motions of religion without any deeply felt conviction. Many students have similar reactions to their schooling, at least at times. At the opposite pole is the feeling of integration, of a powerful bond between one's inner feelings and outward behavior. (An exercise would be to recall experiences in one's own life of alienation and of integration.)

Stripping the word *deviant* of its heavy load of negative emotions may seem easy at first. When one realizes that it usually has extremely strong emotional connotations, then one can use the word in its neutral, sociological sense if one chooses. Actually, the emotional coloring is so strong and so complex that the stripping operation and the dispassionate use of the word is a difficult maneuver. We have all been socialized to feel extremely strong emotions toward deviance and deviants, profound reactions of resentment, fear, and embarrassment. These feelings usually cannot be completely controlled by the desire to be analytic and objective. The sociologist's intent to be dispassionate toward deviance exists in strong tension with his/her inclination to feel the negative emotions of his/her own tribe. Nevertheless, the sociological sense of deviance is still quite different from the ordinary sense of the idea, emotionally, since the tension between neutrality and emotional commitment itself is differentiating. The ordinary member of the tribe feels little or no tension in this respect: his/her condemnation of deviance is wholehearted and un-self-conscious. The sentiment behind "Lock them up in jail and throw away the key" is prevalent, even in those who would not openly endorse such a statement.

There is a third way in which the sociological use of the term *deviance* is different from the conventional usage. The sociological concept of deviance is embedded in a whole set of ideas about the larger system of which deviance is one part. Corresponding to each of these ideas is a set of terms, or nomenclature, for the various parts of the system. We have already used one of these other terms in the discussion, the concept of a social norm. Deviance is an aspect of a larger system that is composed of shared expectations, or norms, on the one hand, and sanctions (rewards and punishments), on the other. Systems of social control exert pressure for conformity to social norms through the operations of sanctions: conformity to shared expectations is rewarded, and nonconformity is punished.

Since the idea of social control provides this book with its principal focus, in the discussion that follows, I provide many examples of the operation of social control. Before doing so, however, I would like to discuss briefly two questions that the reader may have in encountering this argument: What is the purpose of this kind of analysis? The ideas proposed here are certainly awkward, and you say they may be alienating. Why isn't it possible to rely on the experts in our society for approaches to deviance? Professionals such as police and criminologists for crime and psychiatrists and clinical psychologists for mental disorder, drug use, and sexual deviance are in direct contact with the very deviants who are the subjects of this book. Their experience should justify their opinions.

My answer to these questions is in two parts. The first part is that one should not discard the findings and insights that are available in police science, criminology, psychiatry, and clinical psychology. This knowledge, as suggested in the question, is based on intimate and detailed knowledge of deviants and is therefore clearly of great value.

However, and this is a big however, I would also argue that although it is valuable, it is not enough by itself. There is an important bias in the collective wisdom of the professionals who regularly deal with deviants. In some important ways, these professionals are part of the system of social control that is described here. They are not entirely detached investigators of the process of deviance, since they themselves must deal with deviants in ways that are acceptable to the society. A policeman, warden, or clinical psychiatrist or psychologist who merely objectively studies clients would not last long in the job, since it calls, at least in part, for the enforcing of the appropriate social norms. The professionals who deal with deviance, because they are part of the system of social control, usually have a perspective that is, at least in part, congruent with the basic perspective of the particular society they represent. Most prison wardens or psychiatrists are not completely dispassionate about the crimes of their prisoners; they tend to see them, at least in part, as the society does, as abhorrent.

The social control framework offers a more detached and therefore, one hopes, a more objective perspective for examining deviance and the control of deviance. This framework can be applied to deviance in any society, including the society of the analyst. As has already been mentioned, the dispassionate analysis of deviance in one's own society involves the analyst in conflict because of the very basic negative beliefs and feelings shared by all of the members of the society, including the social scientist. But conflict may heighten awareness. This heightening of awareness may be uncomfortable for the analyst but it also increases the objectivity and insightfulness of his/her analysis.

I now return to the concept of a system of social control. As indicated, this system is composed of a very large set of norms, on the one hand, and a set of sanctions, of punishments and rewards, which enforce the norms, on the other. I begin the discussion with a description of social norms. The simplest definition of a norm is a shared expectation, that is, an expectation that is shared by the members of a group. The sense in which an expectation is shared is rather complicated. Social norms can be incredibly rigid and impervious to change, but they can also change overnight. Paradoxically, norms can be both evanescent and unyielding. The great French sociologist Durkheim referred to them as social facts. It is instructive to compare these social facts with physical facts.

There is a sense in which a social fact is enormously more durable than the toughest physical material. The desert tribes who created the Ten Commandments have long since vanished; not a shard remains of their civilization. Yet the moral code they developed is very much alive today, part of the consciousness and behavior of those societies that have a Judeo-Christian heritage. The Ten Commandments survive not merely in the Bible but in our very lives and minds. Shared expectations of this kind are stronger than the strongest steel, more durable than gold.

As I have said, normative codes can collapse and vanish overnight. In any culture, panic and anarchy are unusual but not beyond possibility. More usually, definite change occurs in a measured or gradual way. Changes in shared expectations concerning clothing and appearance are an important part of the phenomenon of fashion. Another example is the pervasive change in language over a much longer time period.

What is the nature of the process of sharing expectations such that norms can be either stronger than steel or weaker than gossamer? Furthermore, what is the relationship of individual expectations to those held by the group? In some instances, it is clear even to individuals strongly opposed to a norm that the norm exists, seemingly independently of their own will or the will of any persons whom they know. As Durkheim indicated, collective representations, or what we call here shared expectations, have exteriority and constraint. They may seem exterior to many or even most of the persons in the society where they obtain, and they are seen, therefore, as constraining on behavior: people actually feel pressure to conform. Durkheim ([1895] 1938) sees norms as so powerful that he gives them a life of their own apart from the people who create them as "partially autonomous realities, with their own way of life." Durkheim does not actually answer the question raised here about the nature of the process involved in the creation and maintenance of shared expectations; he merely suggests that it occurs: "Collective representations are exterior to individual minds. . . . They do not derive from them as such, but from the association of minds, which is a very different thing."

How may one describe the details of the "the association of minds" that Durkheim refers to in a way that makes the exteriority and constraint of norms plausible? This is a crucial question for the understanding of social control. An answer has been suggested by the economist Thomas Schelling (1963). It is instructive to repeat an example he has given of the creation of a shared expectation, in this case, the understanding between the conflicting parties that the Yalu River was to be the boundary of the Korean War:

> If the Yalu River is to be viewed as a limit in the Korean War that was recognized on both sides, its force and authority is to be analyzed not in terms of the joint unilateral recognition of it by both sides of the conflict—not as something that we and the Chinese recognized unilaterally and simultaneously—but as something that we "mutually recognized." It was not just that we recognized it and they recognized it, but that we recognized that they recognized it, they recognized that we recognized it, we recognized that they recognized that we recognized it, and so on. It was a shared expectation. To that extent, it was a

somewhat undeniable expectation. If it commands our attention, then we expect it to be observed and we expect the Chinese to expect us to observe it. We cannot unilaterally detach our expectations from it. In that sense limits and precedents and traditions of this kind have an authority that is not exactly granted to them voluntarily by the participants in a conflict. They acquire magnetism or focal power of their own.

In this example, Schelling (1963) gives what I consider to be an extremely precise definition of a social norm. The people who come to share an expectation need not be in actual contact or consider themselves a group. In this case, the people are at war with each other. But they are sensitive to each other's gestures, so that they "mutually recognize" that they share an expectation. The sharing of the expectation is very deep in that it is not just that the parties all hold the expectation independently, but that each recognizes that the other holds it, and each recognizes that the other recognizes that they hold it, and so on. The parties are not merely in agreement about the Yalu River, they are co-oriented: "I know that you know that I know that if the United States forces go past the river, the Chinese Army will intervene." Another example: "I expect that others will not touch me intimately in public; I assume that most others share this expectation; I assume that most others assume that I share this expectation," etc. A shared expectation exists if there is an infinite series of reciprocating attributions between the members of the group.

As in my definition, Schelling (1963) allows for indefinitely high orders of reciprocating attribution. This allowance evokes Durkheim's exteriority and constraint in its final sentences:

> In that sense limits and precedents and traditions of this kind have an authority that is not exactly granted to them voluntarily by the participants in a conflict. They acquire magnetism or focal power of their own.

The shared expectation is felt as a powerful exterior constraint because each individual agrees, recognizes that his neighbors agree, that they each recognize that he agrees, that he recognizes they recognize, and so on indefinitely. Although he agrees (or disagrees) with the sentiment, it is also something beyond his power to change, or even completely explore. The potentially endless mirror reflections of each of the others' recognitions is felt as something utterly final. From this formulation it follows that each actor feels the presence of expectation with a sense of exteriority and constraint, even if he, as an individual, is himself wholeheartedly dedicated or opposed to the expectation.

To each member of the society, therefore, norms appear to have both an inner reality, a sense of moral obligation and rectitude, and an outer reality, the sense that others are deeply and irrevocably involved in the same moral world as oneself.

The individual's sense of moral coercion from others is complexly determined, because it is in part an assumption, but it is also in part based on reality. One cannot help being aware that others are not indifferent to normative aspects of behavior. Even strangers, when in each other's presence, make subtle but forceful moral claims on each other. The temporary passengers in an elevator inhibit each other's behavior, even to the direction of glance. Most people feel compelled to look at the floor or elevator doors. These inhibitions arise because of actual or expected responses of others to one's behavior, as well as one's own sense of morality.

To put it in a slightly different way, the process of social control involves both control by others and self-control. Self-control operates in two related but different ways. First, the individual can imagine a whole world of response that may never occur. A female college student, considering whether to live with a male friend or not, may suddenly see the issue as her mother may see it—"What would mother think?"—and be guided by her impression of her mother's judgment. Similarly, before standing up in front of the class and giving an answer to a question, a student may consider his answer not only from the professor's point of view but also from that of the class. In some instances, the student refrains from speaking, having imagined how his answer might seem to one or both of these parties.

Second, even real actions of others must be interpreted by the individual as to whether they are responses to the individual's acts, that is, whether they are sanctions. As the student gives an answer in class, he notices that the professor is frowning. The student must decide if the professor's frown is a response to the student's answer. The student remembers that the professor was frowning before the question was asked and decides that the frown is not a response to the answer. The student's interpretation is verified when the professor praises the answer. In the process of social control, sanctions are responses by others to one's behavior. Social control involves imaginative rehearsal and/or interpretation and is therefore in part a process of self-control.

Sanctions may be defined as responses that reward behavior that is seen as conforming to normative expectations (positive sanctions) or punish nonconforming behavior (negative sanctions). That is, they are responses to conformity that bring pleasure to the actor and responses to nonconformity that bring pain. The response need not be extreme and formal, as in the case of a long prison sentence for a major crime; it can be subtle and ephemeral—a frown directed at a speaker with a slight lisp. Social control exerts a powerful force over behavior because the sanctioning process is often continuous and seemingly automatic.

Social control is largely informal. In most instances, it goes on unstated, unseen, and unacknowledged. To be sure, there are important aspects of any system of social control that are formal and explicit. The legal system, both in its criminal and civil sections, and also the disciplinary systems in organizations function in a formal way as a part of social control. Laws, statutes, and codes may serve as explicitly stated norms, and fines, imprisonment, and other disciplinary procedures may serve as sanctions. But the overlap between these formal systems and the larger system of social control in which they play a part is far from complete.

In the first place, the total system of social control in a society is vastly larger than all of the formal systems taken together. In any given society, the total number of laws and codes may be counted in the tens of thousands. The number of formal sanctions is usually extremely small, in the hundreds, perhaps. As suggested in the discussion of the areas of control, in which I consider, as examples, diverse areas such as clothing, language, facial expression, thought, and feeling, the tacit norms and sanctions may come to uncounted millions.

In the second place, the formal systems are not completely accurate indexes of the system of social control. All formal systems contain forms that are not part of functioning system of control—blue-stocking laws, for example, statutes that are unenforced, dead-letter laws. The formal systems stand in relation to a system of social control as dictionaries and grammars stand to a living language: formal description and usage overlap but are distinct entities.

AREAS OF SOCIAL CONTROL

A living language can be considered to arise out of the action of a pervasive system of social control. On the one hand, shared among the speakers are literally millions of expectations concerning grammar, syntax, pronunciation, inflection, gesture, and meaning. On the other hand, a continuous sanctioning process is occurring, in which conformity is rewarded and nonconformity punished. In face-to-face conversation, it is customary for the listener to reward the speaker almost continuously for conformity by looking intently at the speaker, nodding one's head or making some other affirmative gesture, and smiling or at least refraining from frowning. Each of these gestures is a means of communicating to the speaker: "You are doing fine. I am listening. I understand. Please continue." More abstractly, the listener is continually responding to the actions of the speaker with positive sanctions and, in the case of not frowning, with the absence of negative sanctions.

Violation of expectations regarding language, whether verbal or nonverbal, is usually met with misunderstanding or incomprehension at best. Often violations bring responses of ridicule or censure. Adults may censure each other's language violations subtly or diplomatically. Adults with children, or children with children, are much less restrained. The world of the stutterer or the lisper is usually a nightmare of embarrassment.

Group members are extraordinarily sensitive to even slight departures from normative speech expectations. Variations of speech that are extremely slight, such as those due to social class or regional background, will usually produce both real and imagined sanctions. Even a slight residue of working-class inflection from Boston or New Orleans will produce frowns of distaste among middle-class Californians.

As already indicated, clothing and outward physical appearance present another lesson in social control. In modern industrial societies, the rate of change of the fashion in clothing and appearance is much more rapid than fashion in language. Nevertheless, the system of control is equally relentless. As is frequently remarked, even the rebels against the harsh strictures of fashion soon establish their own system of control. The hippie rebellion of the 1960s and the blue-jeaned, T-shirted adolescent of the 1970s quickly developed codes of their own as precise as the ones they rejected. For a teenager at the time of this writing, the choice of fabric, style, and color in buying a pair of Adidas sneakers may be a task requiring excruciating care.

Social control is exercised not only over clothing but also over most other aspects of outward appearance. Hairstyling is an obvious case in point. The length of men's hair usually not only excites responses along an aesthetic dimension but also involves more momentous issues very quickly, as it did both in Cromwell's England and in the 1960s student movement, when it had a political significance. The amount and style of facial cosmetics usually has analogous moral implications for women. In nineteenth-century America, for example, rouge and lipstick were the marks of actresses and prostitutes.

In most societies, fashion in appearance extends to the body itself. The amount of exposure of leg, buttocks, midriff, and bosom is rigidly monitored by custom. Even the shape of the body is not exempt; deformation of the body, especially the bodies of women, is regularly attempted through social control. Their feet have been bound and their lips and buttocks made to protrude by surgery in prior societies. In our own society, injections of silicone are used to shape, lift, and extend the breasts and buttocks, and surgery rejuvenates aging faces and necks. Normative body shapes are rewarded with admiration; non-normative shapes are punished with criticism or neglect.

The relentlessness and pervasiveness of social control over outward forms of behavior and appearance is easily described. But social control does not stop with outer forms; it penetrates deeply into the inner life of thought and feeling. I begin this discussion with the issue of control over facial expression, since facial expression partakes of both outer and inner worlds. There are many situations in which facial expression is clearly subject to social control. At a funeral or at a school examination, a smile may bring an open rebuke just as a frown may receive a similar response at a cocktail party. In the large cities in modern society, a norm governing facial expression in public appears to be developing: it requires an expression signaling no emotion.

Some of the humor and apprehension generated by the film *Invasion of the Body Snatchers* rests on this issue: that the blankness of the zombies in the San Francisco locale only slightly exaggerates the behavior that is becoming the norm in real life.

The expectation that the public facial expression on a metropolitan street will be an emotionless mask presumably shows social control only over the outward expression of feeling. Often, however, social control extends to the actual feeling within. For example, in most human groups, to feel either too much or too little grief is to be subjected to negative sanctions. A person who feels little or no grief over the death of a parent would be considered a moral monster. On the other hand, the widow who mourns too long over her dead spouse will be rebuked. She may be told that she is being "morbid." In instances such as these, it is not merely outward expression that is being controlled but especially and mainly inner feeling. As Arlie Hochschild (1979) has indicated, we expend considerable effort doing "emotion work," that is, struggling either to evoke a feeling that our culture deems appropriate or suppressing a feeling that it deems inappropriate. In modern societies, the bride and bridegroom are expected to feel love for each other, although such an expectation is a comparatively recent event in human history. In all societies in human history, it would appear that social control exerts intense pressure on members to hate their tribal or national enemies, especially in times of conflict or war. Much the same can be said for persons defined as internal enemies, such as minorities and deviants. As I suggest, the extremely strong negative feelings mobilized by acts of deviance, especially moral outrage and indignation, are a centrally important aspect of the social control of deviance.

Like feelings, thoughts and beliefs are aspects of the inner life that seem private, yet like feelings they are also subject to the action of social control. Before Magellan, anyone who thought that the Earth might not be flat would have been considered insane. Similarly, in the 1960s and most of the 1970s, activists who thought that the FBI and CIA were doing what they were actually doing were considered paranoid. The thoughts and beliefs of children are rigorously subject to control. For example, when my oldest child was about 4 years old, he went through a period of nightmares about ghosts and threatening animals that would wake him from sleep. Like any other upstanding member of the tribe, I hastened to assure him that the images he had seen in his sleep were not real. (One incident occurred when I was reassuring him after he had awakened from an animal dream. He pointed to a fold in the bedclothes, asking what it was. I said, "That's just the sheet." Only half awake, he shouted in terror: "A sheep! A sheep!") At about the same time, he and I were involved in a protracted struggle over the cleanliness of his hands at mealtime. Whenever I asked him to wash his hands, he would inspect them, then show them to me:

Son: They are not dirty, they're clean.
Father: But they may have germs on them.

At this remark, he would again inspect his hands:

Son: I don't see any germs.
Father: You can't see them, they're too little.

After considerable time, effort, and emotion, I succeeded in convincing my young son that the dream images he had actually seen were not real and the germs that he had never seen were. I had functioned as an agent of social control over his beliefs about reality. Yet in most societies in human history, the situation would have been reversed. The images in the dream would have been considered real, manifestations of the night-wandering spirits of the dead, whereas the germs on the hands, unseen, would have been considered unreal. To a large extent, the system of social control in a society constructs reality for its members. As shown in Chapter 4, the social construction of reality is a central issue in the sociological approach to mental disorder.

To review so far: All human groups have a system of social control that shapes all areas of experience—behavior, perception, thought, and feeling. This system operates to obtain conformity: acts that meet normative expectations are positively sanctioned, and acts that violate normative expectations are negatively sanctioned. The system acts through both actual sanctions and through those imagined or assumed. Indeed, the imagined responses of others to one's acts are probably fully as important as their real responses in the operation of social control. In becoming adult members of the tribe, children quickly learn to forestall punishment and gain reward from others by rehearsing their acts in their imagination. In order to imagine accurately other's responses, the child learns probable viewpoints of others in the society, at least in part. In this process of socialization, self-control becomes a crucial aspect of social control.

Although social control works relentlessly, both within and without, to shape behavior, perception, thought, and feeling, its actions are not automatic and inevitable. Indeed, in any given situation, there is some uncertainty not only as to whether others will respond with sanctions to a given act, but even as to what the relevant expectations are. In real life, the provenance of norms and sanctions is a matter of interpretation and negotiation. In most situations, the police seem to believe and act as if they have considerable discretion in deciding whether or not a crime has been committed. Police may define behavior that could be seen as vandalism as a prank: "Boys will be boys." Furthermore, if they decide that a crime has been committed, they seem to believe and act as if they had considerable discretion to decide whether or not to sanction the purported offender. Relentlessly as it may seem to function when viewed abstractly, in any given situation, the operation of social control has a probabilistic and indeterminate character. This indeterminate character of social control is an essential feature and provides, therefore, considerable matter for deliberation for potential offenders, agents of social control, and for scholars of deviance.

To be sure, one can imagine instances where the ambiguity of the system is vanishingly small. If I seek to remove the gold from Fort Knox by stealth or force of arms, the likelihood that my action, if detected, would not be defined as a violation or not sanctioned negatively may be infinitesimally small. However, it is not inconceivable. For example, it is unlikely, but not impossible, that my action may be defined as an act of national liberation. Needless to say, the odds at this particular moment may be astronomically long. The point is that since the operation of social control involves human beings with the capacity for interpreting and negotiating, there is always an element of uncertainty. To put it in a somewhat different way, each time a shared conformity to expectation is upheld by positive sanctioning or nonconformity is punished, the system of social control is affirmed anew. A social order is stable insofar as it receives continuous affirmation in the lives and actions of its members. At any moment, such affirmation may cease. When it does, the order will change or even disappear. Involvement in a social order requires the continual re-creation of that order by its members.

There is an implication of the idea of the indeterminacy of social control that the reader, in his or her capacity as a member of the tribe, may find hard to accept. Crimes and other normative violations are not only relative to the moral order of a particular tribe. The moral order itself is not absolute and fixed but subject to pervasive and continuous testing, in every act, thought, and feeling of its members. Just as the moral order is continually created anew, so every deviant act is a creation, not only of the deviant but also of those who interpret his or her behavior as deviant. Categories of deviance are not absolute: There is no such thing as crime per se or, as shown in the chapter on mental illness, psychiatric symptoms per se. The actions that are categorized in this way are selected by each society somewhat differently and in each concrete instance within a given society are interpreted and negotiated anew.

The philosopher Kant said: "Two things fill the mind with awe: the starry sky above and the moral law within." The process of social control, of which the "the moral law within" is a part, is itself an awesome and improbable phenomenon. Its operation is usually pervasive, relentless, and invisible, capable of stability for millennia, and equally capable of gradual or instantaneous change. Our discussion now turns to the operation of social control in one particular area, the control of deviance.

THE SOCIETAL REACTION TO DEVIANCE

As already indicated, the concept of deviance is widely used in social science to mean violations of normative expectations that are likely to bring responses of indignation and moral outrage from members of the tribe. In this usage, therefore, most normative violations are not seen as instances of deviance. Although belching at a formal dinner would certainly be impolite and would elicit some moral outrage in Western societies, it would not be considered deviant behavior of the level of other violations such as murder, treason, or incest. In some Bedouin societies, however, it is not only polite but expected.

How does one draw the line to distinguish between deviance and other violations? In this discussion, I follow the usage that deviance is a normative violation that may obtain all three of the following responses: moral outrage or *stigma, segregation,* and *labeling.* The possibility that these three responses will follow a violation can be used to define deviance.

In this discussion, I argue that stigma is the single most important aspect of the societal reaction to deviance, and that it is also the most intricate. The dimensions of the other two components are straightforward. Segregation implies special procedures for deviants: prisons, asylums, criminal courts, commitment hearings, drunk tanks. All societies have a particular status reserved for deviants and formal procedures for demoting offenders into that status and for promoting them back into the status of normal members of society. We return to this issue in the discussion of status lines.

Labeling, in the sense that it is used here, is one particular aspect of the process of the segregation of deviants into a special status. By virtue of the special procedures of segregation, the offender receives an official label (e.g., thief, convict, schizophrenic, mental patient, prostitute). These labels or status names are also related to stigmatization, however, since they always carry a heavy weight of moral condemnation.

At the core of the societal reaction to deviance is the process of stigmatization. Deviance is behavior that arouses extraordinarily strong collective loathing. A deviant is that person whose normative violations have aroused strong emotions in the other members of the society. In the process of labeling, this moral opprobrium somehow becomes attached to the deviant; he or she is stigmatized.

In order to understand the societal reaction, it is necessary to realize that the emotional reaction to deviance is usually in excess of the appropriate response. I call this excess, which may be quite small or very large, the surplus emotional response. Stigma occurs because of the surplus.

How is it possible to speak of a surplus emotional response? There is a difficult judgment involved, because there is always a component of the emotional response to deviance that is appropriate. A social order is built upon predictable behavior. Unpredictable behavior often brings social trans-actions to a standstill and therefore gives rise to fear and anger. Consider one of the rules of the road, "Stay on the right side of the road." There is nothing inherently correct about the right side of the road. The left would do equally well, as it does in England. Once chosen, however, it becomes sacrosanct. The social system of the highways does not work perfectly or even very well, since there are many collisions. Nevertheless, driving on the wrong side of the road is a normative violation that brings very strong negative emotions of anger and fear: "You crazy son-of-a-bitch, you're trying to kill me!" The shared expectations of the highway bring some predictability to behavior and therefore a measure of safety.

Oddly enough, the repeated violation of the highway code, even though it may have deadly results, is not highly stigmatized. In the United States, at least, the societal reaction to violations of the rules of the road, rather than arousing an excess emotional response, does the opposite. There seems to be a deficit rather than a surplus emotional response. The punishment of traffic violations is notoriously light compared with other kinds of offenses of com-parable harm or injury. Perhaps, like homicide in Roman law, middle-class people are protected from offenses that they are likely to perpetrate. It is sig-nificant that there is no vernacular label, a short and opprobrious epithet, comparable to thief or whore, for the long-term traffic offender.

On the other hand, there are the stigmatized offenses, such as those against person or property, the rules of reality, sobriety, and sexual propriety. There is always a label, both official and vernacular, for these violators and for their violations. These labels are surface manifestation of a deep and intense emo-tional response involving fear, anger, and/or embarrassment. Why these par-ticular emotions? One reason for fear arousal has already been indicated in the discussion of the rules of the road. Normative behavior gives rise to a pre-dictable world in a very concrete and practical way. Adherence to conven-tions of speech, dress, and facial expression allows each of us to collaborate with others with a minimum of effort and conflict. Suppose you are walking by yourself in a secluded section of a park in a strange city. If you meet a stranger who is bizarrely dressed, speaks in an odd way, and/or shows a facial expression that seems inappropriate to the context, you would probably be frightened because you would not know what to expect. On the other hand, the same stranger in the same situation, if he is conforming in dress, speech, and facial expression may not be particularly fearful. Every item of dress, word, and fleeting facial expression brings reassurance of predictability.

There is another way in which normative violations generate fear that is somewhat different from the simple issue of the predictability of specific ac-tions. As already indicated, most of the reality of the world that is experienced by human beings is socially constructed. Wholesale violations of social norms shatter this world. In a racist society, any perturbation of the color line may be experienced as cataclysmic. There is a sense of shock, at least initially, even when the violations are local and temporary. For me, the first few days of driving on the left side of the road in England has a nightmare quality. Violations of constitutive social norms give rise to ontological fear, that is, the fear that reality itself is collapsing.

The explanation of the emotions of anger and resentment that deviance arouses corresponds to the link between unpredictability and fear previously discussed. Unpredictability gives rise not only to danger but also to frustration. It is difficult to get through a social transaction with a person who is breaking the rules. Frustration is the basic context for anger and resentment, particularly where there is even a suspicion that the frustration is intentional. Most members of the tribe, most of the time, suspect that deviance is willed. Anger is the result.

Explaining the function of the emotion of embarrassment that arises in connection with deviance is less obvious. Embarrassment usually arises in contexts where a person loses face in public. Humiliation is a very strong form of the same emotion. It is easy to see that the rule breaker herself would be embarrassed, even if she is the only one who perceives her gaffe, as suggested in the quotation from Bell concerning inappropriate clothing. But what about the others who witness the rule violation? Why should they be embarrassed? The answer to this question is not at all obvious.

One reason is that persons who are cooperating with each other in managing a social transaction necessarily and inevitably identify with each other. Suppose I am involved with another person in lifting a table. In order to coordinate our actions, I must see the whole transaction not only from my point of view but from the other person's as well. This kind of identification is not moral and empathic, at least not in the first instance. It is simply practical. To understand the speech of another person, even if I happen to dislike that person with great intensity, I necessarily must take that person's point of view, to locate myself with respect to that person's position, to grasp the meaning of the speech. This kind of process is referred to as role-taking and is thought to be the basis of interaction between human beings that is distinctively social. The idea of social norm as an infinite series of shared attributions predicates role-taking.

Given the phenomenon of role-taking, the basis of embarrassment over deviance by onlookers can be grasped. Onlookers are embarrassed over acts of deviance because they almost automatically identify with other members of the tribe. Perhaps it is for this reason that most people conspire to avoid embarrassing others, generating tact about tact. It is not merely kindness but self-protection. Embarrassment is extremely painful to witness: blushing, averting the gaze, looking at the floor, wishing to escape the scene yet feeling paralyzed and shamed. The pain can be direct for oneself or vicarious for another.

But there is a more fundamental reason for embarrassment and shame responses in the societal reaction. The rules of behavior that govern social interaction are not only exterior to us. In our socialization, they become part of us, our second nature. They make up a substantial part of each self. For this reason, deviance is personally offensive; we feel wounded and betrayed by it. The multiform contracts for behavior and being that each of us has entered into are thrashed by deviants. Criminal deviance announces that the legal order that we accept as part of the natural state of things is not sacrosanct. The behavior of the "mentally ill," similarly, announces that the emotional/relational world is also not inviolable; it violates the emotional/relational status quo. This issue will be considered in the next chapter, which translates the symptoms of mental disorder into "residual deviance," the breaking of taken-for-granted rules.

One direction that the societal reaction takes is humiliated fury. Those persons whose sense of self is insecure may react violently and irrationally to the threat of crime or mental disorder. Their moral order has been violated, and someone must pay. Persons in the grip of humiliated fury become obsessed with controlling or punishing those are who are seen as a threat to their moral order. By projecting the entire problem onto others, rather than also facing their own shame and insecurity, they escape from increasing their own self-awareness. The pain of shame and embarrassment is an important aspect of the emotional response to deviance as are the emotions of anger and fear.

At least a part of the emotional response to deviance is usually displaced onto the deviants from other areas of the individual's life. Deviants (and enemies and strangers, as well) are heirs to our childhood fears of the bogeyman, of the dark, of all that is unknown and menacing. It is this displacement of emotion that gives rise to the indelibility of stigma and to many of the other peculiarities of the societal reaction.

It long has been observed that there is a cycle in the societal reaction to deviance that contains three phases: quiescence, exposé, reform or repression, followed by a repetition of the cycle (Lemert 1951, pp. 55–64). Public attention to prisons and mental hospitals is particularly marked by this cycle, but it can also be observed in the cycle of police attention to drunks and vice. This cycle is difficult to understand on rational grounds, since reasonable attempts to solve outstanding social problems would be marked by a more or less constant level of concern and attention. When based on irrational emotions, however, responses are apt to be too little or too much. That is, these emotions are denied until some shocking event necessitates action. When this occurs, there is usually an overreaction, a hysterical outburst of concern. The denial of emotion corresponds to the phase of quiescence; the second phase, the exposé, is the trigger for the last phase, the hysterical overkill of the phase of reform or repression.

The effects of the surplus emotional response to deviance can also be seen in another way. The indelibility of stigma results from the surplus, since it is displaced and therefore quite irrational. The formal structure of retribution or treatment never quite removes all the stigma; the ex-offender or ex–mental patient who has "served his time" or been "cured" still carries some of the stigma of deviance in most cases. The irrational component of stigma also helps explain the cyclical character of the societal reaction. Really effective reform is difficult to mobilize because formally designated deviants are tainted by stigma: their cause is subtly discounted in the political process. A flagrant version of this process can be seen in public reaction to gangland killings: "Let them kill each other off." But it also applies, in a more subtle way, to all societal responses to deviance.

Another example of the discounting process can be seen in some remarks once made to me by a member of the Chamber of Deputies in Italy. This deputy was describing some of the notorious flaws in the mental health system in Italy. When I asked him why there were no reform bills in the chamber, he said: "No one wants to defend the mentally ill. In Italy they are called 'pazzi.' If I were to initiate a reform law, my opponents would say, that I am pazzo too" (at this point he makes a circular motion with his index finger pointed at his temple). The mentally ill are so tainted emotionally that their taint may rub off on their protectors. For this reason, it is difficult to mount a rational program for the management of deviance. Most programs are marked either by impulsive action, on the one hand, or by pretense, on the other, corresponding to the hysterical or to the denial phase in the dynamics of collective emotion.

As can be seen quickly from the preceding discussion, some of the ideas used in outlining the social control of deviance are vague and elusive. It is easy to point to the procedures and labels used in the segregation of formally certified deviants. But where do we find the emotional responses that have been emphasized in this discussion? How can one tell if there is a surplus emotional response or a deficit? Similarly in the discussion of the normative system, one can easily locate and list laws and codes that are part of the formal system. But how can one find the unwritten rules and the unstated codes?

These are important questions, and they are difficult to answer. Investigations of these issues are occurring at the frontier of social science and psychology. A very conservative position to take would be that until there is a wealth of agreed-upon facts about these matters, they should be left out of the reckoning. I take an alternative position. All of us act upon our understanding of emotional responses and unstated rules everyday. This discussion will appeal to the untutored intuition of the reader. To be competent in social interaction, one must be an "expert" in these matters, although one's expertise is so taken for granted that it is hardly ever acknowledged. I believe the conservative position on evidence and fact in social science is a useful strategy for research and teaching, but it is quite incomplete. To rely completely on formal, stated knowledge in social science is to make us foreigners in our own country, having only textbook knowledge of the language and the customs, and therefore really not understanding even the simplest social transaction, let alone the more complex and subtle ones. This book will appeal to both scientific knowledge and to the reader's intuition in order to convey a sophisticated understanding of deviance and social control.

CONCLUSION

In the preceding discussion, the theory of the social control of deviant behavior has been outlined. The theory posits a system for obtaining conforming behavior that is unique to each particular society. The principal components of the system are a vast set of norms that are supported by sanctions. Deviance in a particular system is those normative violations that arouse public outrage and can result in segregation and labeling of the offenders. Finally, the procedures for segregation and labeling result in a status line that divides offenders from nonoffenders. The concept of the status line suggests a way of interpreting the causation and management of deviance that is alternative to perspectives that focus on individuals.

What is the advantage of the social control perspective? Is it anything more than a new set of special terms? One advantage has already been suggested in using special terms. Concepts like social control, norms, and deviance help the analyst to disengage from the culture-bound perspective of the society being studied. They are general terms applicable to any society, so that comparisons are made easily. Furthermore, these terms help to detach the argument from the emotional values of a particular society, so that objectivity is increased.

There is a second advantage that has not been mentioned yet in this discussion. The social control perspective is much broader than the individual perspective in that it does not prejudge in conflicts between individual deviants and society. The individual perspective suggests two questions: What causes deviance? and How can it be stopped? These are important questions, but they do not exhaust the kinds of questions that should be asked about deviance. There are historical questions concerning social control: Why does a particular society define as deviant a behavior that another society does not? For example, the individual perspective does not exhaust the issue of marijuana use in our era. Why do young people smoke marijuana, and how can it be stopped? A more interesting question is, Who opposes marijuana use, and why is this opposition so strong? Why is marijuana use more severely penalized than the use of alcohol and tranquilizers? The social control perspective calls attention to the system of norms and sanctions as well as to the offenders and their offenses.

One tactic in understanding deviance concerns broad classes of deviance. As suggested in later chapters, crime is produced by criminals, but it is also produced by legislatures. If a legislature were to change the laws governing corporation violations and other "white-collar" crimes to criminal, rather than civil actions, it could create thousands of criminals overnight. A move in the opposite direction is currently happening in psychiatry: It has been agreed that homosexuality is not a mental illness. To the extent that this new definition is accepted by psychiatrists and other key societal agents, thousands of homosexuals will be promoted out of their deviant status.

The social control perspective can also be applied to particular cases of deviance. Why are some offenders detected and punished and others ignored? This is the basic question asked by the "labeling" approach to deviance. This approach is concerned with the contingencies that give rise to status demotion for some offenders and not for others. It is also concerned with the effects of segregation, labeling, and stigma on "chronicity" (i.e., on the stability of rule-breaking behavior). During one point in English history, a man convicted of theft was branded with an F (for felon) on his forehead. This action ensured a career of robbery, since a person so branded could never obtain honest employment. This was an extreme instance of the way in which the societal reaction to deviance produced further deviance. The labeling approach concerns the ways in which society produces deviance, sometimes in ways that are considerably more subtle than branding. Jerome Frank (1961), among others, has addressed this issue as it concerns mental illness:

> By teaching people to regard certain types of distress or behavioral oddities as illnesses rather than as normal reactions to life's stresses, harmless eccentricities, or moral weaknesses, it may cause alarm and increase the demand for psychotherapy. This may explain the curious fact that the use of psychotherapy tends to keep pace with its availability. The greater the number of treatment facilities and the more widely they are known, the larger the number of persons seeking their help. Psychotherapy is the only form of treatment that at least to some extent, appears to create the illness it treats. (pp. 6–7)

As is the case with most other areas of human behavior, our understanding of deviance is at a very elementary level. The social control perspective offers the opportunity for broadening the level of analysis and therefore of increasing our awareness in a complex and confusing area of inquiry.

4

Residual Deviance

One source of immediate embarrassment to any social theory of "mental illness" is that the terms used in referring to these phenomena in our society prejudge the issue. The medical metaphor "mental illness" suggests a determinate process that occurs within the individual: the unfolding and development of disease. In order to avoid this assumption, we will utilize sociological, rather than medical concepts to formulate the problem. Particularly crucial to the formulation of the problem is the idea of psychiatric "symptoms," which is applied to the behavior that is taken to signify the existence of an underlying mental illness. Since in the great majority of cases of mental illness, the existence of this underlying illness is unproved, we need to discuss "symptomatic" behavior in terms that do not involve the assumption of illness.

Two concepts seem to be suited best to the task of discussing psychiatric symptoms from a sociological point of view: rule-breaking and deviance. Rule-breaking refers to behavior that is in clear violation of the agreed-upon rules of the group. These rules are usually discussed by sociologists as social norms. If the symptoms of mental illness are to be construed as violations of social norms, it is necessary to specify the type of norms involved. Most norm violations do not cause the violator to be labeled as mentally ill, but as ill-mannered, ignorant, sinful, criminal, or perhaps just harried, depending on the type of norm involved. There are innumerable norms, however, over which consensus is so complete that the members of a group appear to take them for granted. A host of such norms surrounds even the simplest conversation: a person engaged in conversation is expected to face toward his partner, rather than directly away from him; if his gaze is toward the partner, he is expected to look toward the other's eyes, rather than, say, toward his forehead; to stand at a proper conversational distance, neither one inch away nor across the room, and so on. A person who regularly violated these expectations probably would not be thought to be merely ill-bred, but as strange, bizarre, and frightening, because his behavior violates the assumptive world of the group, the world that is construed to be the only one that is natural, decent, and possible.

The concept of deviance used here will follow Becker's (1963) usage. He argues that deviance can be most usefully considered as a quality of people's response to an act, rather than as a characteristic of the act itself:

> Social groups create deviance by making the rules whose infraction constitutes deviance, and by applying those rules to particular people and labeling them as outsiders. . . . [D]eviance is not a quality of the act the person commits, but rather a consequence of the application by others of rules and sanctions to an "offender." The deviant is one to whom that label has successfully been applied; deviant behavior is behavior that people so label. (p. 9)

By this definition, deviants are not a group of people who have committed the same act, but are a group of people who have been stigmatized as deviants.

Becker argues that the distinction between rule-breaking and deviance is necessary for scientific purposes:

> Since deviance is, among other things, a consequence of the responses of others to a person's act, students of deviance cannot assume that they are dealing with a homogeneous category when they study people who have been labeled deviant. That is, they cannot assume that these people have actually . . . broken some rule, because the process of labeling may not be infallible. . . . Furthermore, they cannot assume that the category of those labeled deviant will contain all those who actually have broken a rule, for many offenders may escape apprehension and thus fail to be included in the population of "deviants" they study. Insofar as the category lacks homogeneity and fails to include all the cases that belong in it, one cannot reasonably expect to find common factors of personality or life situation that will account for the supposed deviance. (p. 9)

For the purpose of this discussion, we will conform to Becker's separation of rule-breaking and deviance. Rule-breaking will refer to a class of acts, violations of social norms, and deviance to particular acts that have been publicly and officially labeled as norm violations.

Using Becker's distinction, we can categorize most psychiatric symptoms as instances of residual rule-breaking or residual deviance. The culture of the group provides a vocabulary of terms for categorizing many norm violations: crime, perversion, drunkenness, and bad manners are familiar examples. Each of these terms is derived from the type of norm broken and, ultimately, from the type of behavior involved. After exhausting these categories, however, there is always a residue of the most diverse kinds of violations for which the culture provides no explicit label. For example, although there is great cultural variation in what is defined as decent or real, each culture tends to reify its definition of decency and reality and so provides no way of handling violations of its expectations in these areas. The typical norm governing decency or reality, therefore, literally "goes without saying," and its violation is unthinkable for most of its members. For the convenience of the society in construing those instances of unnamable rule-breaking that are called to its attention, these violations may be lumped together into a residual category: witchcraft, spirit possession, or, in our own society, mental illness. In this discussion, the diverse kinds of rule-breaking for which our society provides no explicit label and that therefore sometimes lead to the labeling of the violator as mentally ill, will be considered to be technically *residual rule-breaking*.

Let us consider further some of the implications of a definition of psychiatric "symptoms" as instances of residual deviance. In *Behavior in Public Places*, Goffman (1964) develops the idea that there is a complex of social norms that regulate the way in which a person may behave when in the presence, or potentially in the presence, of other persons. Goffman's discussion of the norms regarding "involvements," particularly, illustrates how such psychiatric symptoms as withdrawal and hallucinations may be regarded as violations of residual rules.

Noting that lolling and loitering are usually specifically prohibited in codes of law, Goffman goes on to point out that there is a much more elaborate set of norms centering around the expectation that a person appearing in public should be involved or engaged in doing something:

> The rule against "having no purpose," or being disengaged, is evident in the exploitation of untaxing involvements to rationalize or mask desired lolling—a way of covering one's physical presence in a situation with a veneer of acceptable visible activity. Thus when individuals want a "break" in their work routine, they may remove themselves to a place where it is acceptable to smoke and there smoke in a pointed fashion. Certain minimal "recreational" activities are also used as covers for disengagement, as in the case of "fishing" off river banks where it is guaranteed that no fish will disturb one's reverie, or "getting a tan" on the beach—activity that shields reverie or sleep, although, as with hoboes' lolling, a special uniform may have to be worn, which proclaims and institutionalizes the relative inactivity. As might be expected, when the context firmly provides a dominant involvement that is outside the situation, as when

riding in a train or airplane, then gazing out the window, or reverie, or sleeping may be quite permissible. In short, the more the setting guarantees that the participant has not withdrawn from what he ought to be involved in, the more liberty it seems he will have to manifest what would otherwise be considered withdrawal in the situation. (1964, pp. 58–59)

The rule requiring that an adult be "involved" when in public view is unstated in our society, yet so taken for granted that individuals almost automatically shield their lack of involvement in socially acceptable ways, as illustrated in the quotation. Thus the rule of involvement would seem to be a residual rule.

Two types of involvements that Goffman discusses are particularly relevant to a discussion of residual deviance: "away" and "occult involvements." "Away" is described in this manner:

While outwardly participating in an activity within a social situation, an individual can allow his attention to turn from what he and everyone else considered the real or serious world, and give himself up for a time to a play-like world in which he alone participates. This kind of inward emigration from the gathering may be called "away," and we find that strict regulations obtain regarding it. Perhaps the most important kind of away is that through which the individual relives some past experiences or rehearses some future ones, this taking the form of what is variously called reverie, brown study, woolgathering, daydreaming or autistic thinking. At such times the individual may demonstrate his absence from the current situation by a preoccupied, faraway look in his eyes, or by a sleeplike stillness of his limbs, or by that special class of side involvements that can be sustained in an utterly "unconscious" abstracted manner—humming, doodling, drumming the fingers on a table, hair twisting, nose picking, scratching. (1964, pp. 69–70)

This discussion is relevant to the psychiatric symptoms that come under the rubric of "withdrawal," showing that the behavior that is called withdrawal in itself is not socially unacceptable. An "away" is met with public censure only when it occurs in a socially unacceptable context. But this is to say that there are residual rules governing the context in which "aways" may take place. When an "away" violates these rules, it is apt to be called "withdrawal" and taken as evidence of mental illness.

"Occult involvement" is defined as a subtype of "awayness":

There is a kind of awayness where the individual gives others the impression, whether warranted or not, that he is not aware that he is "away." This is the area of what psychiatry terms "hallucinations" and delusionary states. Corresponding to these "unnatural" verbal activities, there are unnatural bodily ones, where the individual's activity is patiently task-like but not "understandable" or "meaningful." The unnatural action may even involve the holding or grasping of something, as when an adult mental patient retains a tight hold on a doll or a fetish-like piece of cloth. Here the terms "mannerism," "ritual act," or "posturing" are applied, which, like the term "unnatural," are clear enough in their way but hardly tell us with any specificity what it is that characterizes "natural" acts. (1964, pp. 75–76)

At first glance, it would seem that if there were ever a type of behavior that in itself would be seen as abnormal, it would be "occult involvements." As Goffman notes, however, there is an element of cultural definition even with "occult involvements": "There are societies in which conversation with a spirit not present is as acceptable when sustained by properly authorized persons as is conversation over a telephone in American society" (1964:79). Furthermore, he points out that even in American society, there are occasions in which "occult involvement" is not censured: "Those who attend a seance would not consider it inappropriate for the medium to interact with 'someone on the other side,' whether they believe this to be staged or a genuine interaction. And certainly we define praying as acceptable when done at proper occasions" (1964, p. 79). Thus, talking to spirits and praying to God are not improper in themselves; indeed, they are seen as legitimate modes of activity when they follow the proprieties—that is, when they occur in the socially proper circumstances and are conducted by persons recognized as legitimately, even though occultly, involved.

Two significant implications follow from this discussion of the etiquette of involvement. The first is that such psychiatric symptoms as withdrawal, hallucinations, continual muttering, and posturing may be categorized as violations of certain social norms—those norms so taken for granted that they are not explicitly verbalized, which we have called residual rules. In particular instances discussed here, the residual rule concerned involvement in public places. It is true, of course, that various specific aspects of the involvement rule occasionally are found, for example, in books of etiquette. Here, for example, is a typical proscription concerning involvement with one's own person in public places:

> Men should never look in the mirror nor comb their hair in public. At most a man may straighten his necktie and smooth his hair with his hand. It is probably unnecessary to add that it is most unattractive to scratch one's head, to rub one's face or touch one's teeth, or to clean one's fingernails in public. All these things should be done privately. (Fenwick 1948, p. 11; quoted in Goffman 1964)

Although we could point to many such informal rules, it is important to note that they are all situationally specific. There is nowhere codified a general principle of involvement or even self-involvement. Unlike codified principles, such as the Ten Commandments, it is one of those expectations that it is felt should govern the behavior of every decent person, even though it goes unsaid. Because it goes unsaid, we are not equipped by our culture to smoothly categorize violations of such a rule but rather may resort to a residual catchall category of violations (i.e., symptoms of mental illness).

This idea points to the profoundly conservative tendency of the current conception of mental illness. By putting the causes of residual deviance inside the deviant, it protects the current emotional/relational status quo. Since most people are highly invested in this realm and unwilling to countenance it, the concept of mental illness offers them a way of avoiding considering the quality of their feelings and relationships.

If it proves to be correct that most symptoms of mental illness can be systematically classified as violations of culturally particular normative networks, then these symptoms may be removed from the realm of universal physical events, where they now tend to be placed by psychiatric theory, along with other culture-free symptoms such as fever, and may be investigated sociologically and anthropologically like any other item of social behavior.

A second implication of the redefinition of psychiatric symptoms as residual deviance is the great emphasis that this perspective puts on the context in which the "symptomatic" behavior occurs. As Goffman repeatedly shows, "aways," "occult involvements," and other kinds of rule violations do not in themselves bring forth censure; it is only when socially unqualified persons perform these acts or perform them in inappropriate contexts. That is, these acts are objectionable when they occur in a manner that does not conform to the unstated, but nevertheless operative etiquette that governs them. Although recently psychiatric discussions of symptomatology have begun to display considerable interest in the social context, it is still true that psychiatric diagnosis tends to focus on the pattern of symptomatic behavior itself, to the neglect of the context in which the symptom occurs. The significance of this tendency in psychiatric diagnostic procedures is discussed later.[1]

The remainder of this chapter is devoted to a discussion of the origins, prevalence, and course of the behavior that we have defined here as residual rule-breaking.

THE ORIGINS OF RESIDUAL RULE-BREAKING

It is customary in psychiatric research to seek a single generic source or at best a small number of sources for mental illness. The redefinition of psychiatric symptoms as residual deviance immediately suggests, however, that there should be an unlimited number of sources of deviance. The first proposition follows.

Proposition 1:   *Residual rule-breaking arises from fundamentally diverse sources.*

Four distinct types of sources are discussed here: organic, psychological, external stress, and volitional acts of innovation or defiance. The organic and psychological origins of residual rule-breaking are widely noted and are not discussed at length here. It has been demonstrated repeatedly that particular cases of mental disorder had their origin in genetic, biochemical, or physiological conditions. Psychological sources are also frequently indicated: peculiarity of upbringing and training have been reported often, particularly in the psychoanalytic literature. The great majority of precise and systematic studies of causation of mental disorder have been limited to either organic or psychological sources.

It is widely granted, however, that psychiatric symptoms can also arise from external stress: from drug ingestion, from the sustained fear and hardship of combat, and from deprivation of food, sleep, and even sensory experience. Excerpts from reports on the consequences of stress will illustrate the rule-breaking behavior that is generated by this less familiar source.

Physicians have long known that toxic substances can cause psychotic-like symptoms when ingested in appropriate doses. A wide variety of substances have been the subject of experimentation in producing "model psychoses." Drugs such as a mescaline and LSD-25, particularly, have been described as producing fairly close replicas of psychiatric symptoms, such as visual hallucinations, loss of orientation to space and time, and interference with thought processes. Here is an excerpt from a report by a qualified psychologist who had taken LSD-25:

> One concomitant of LSD that I shared with other subjects was distortion of the time sense. The subjective clock appeared to race. This was observed even at 25 milligrams in counting 60 seconds. My tapping rate was also speeded up. On the larger dose (1/2 gram) my time sense was displaced by hours. I thought the afternoon was well spent when it was only 1:00 P.M. I could look at my watch and realize the error, but I continued to be disoriented in time. The time sense depends on the way time is "filled," and I was probably responding to the quickened tempo of experience.
>
> This was in fact, my overwhelming impression of LSD. Beginning with the physiological sensations (lightheartedness, excitement) I was shortly flooded by a montage of ideas, images, and feelings that seemed to thrust themselves upon me unbidden. I had glimpses of very bright thoughts, like a fleeting insight into the psychotic process, which I wanted to write down. But they pushed each other aside. Once gone, they could not be recaptured because the parade of new images could not be stopped. (C. C. Bennett 1960, pp. 606–607)

The time disorientation described is a familiar psychiatric symptom, as is the ideational "pressure," which is usually described as a feature of manic excitement.

Combat psychosis and psychiatric symptoms arising from starvation have been repeatedly described in the psychiatric literature. Psychotic symptoms resulting from sleeplessness are less familiar. One instance is used to illustrate this reaction. Brauchi and West (1961, p. 11) reported the symptoms of two participants in a radio marathon that required them to talk alternately every 30 minutes. After 168 hours, one of the contestants felt that he and his opponent belonged to a secret club of nonsleepers. He accused his girlfriend of kissing an observer, even though she was with him at the time. He felt he was being punished, had transient auditory and visual hallucinations, and became suggestible, he and his opponent exhibiting a period of *folie a deux* when the delusions and hallucinations of the one were accepted by the other. He showed persistence of his psychotic symptoms, with delusions about secret agents, and felt that he was responsible for the Israel-Egypt conflict. His reactions contain many elements that psychiatrists would describe as paranoid and depressive features.

A number of studies have shown that deprivation of sensory stimulation can cause hallucinations and other symptoms. In one such study, Heron (1961) reported on subjects who were cut off from sensations:

> Male college students were paid to lie 24 hours a day on a comfortable bed in a lighted semi-soundproof cubicle . . . wearing translucent goggles which admitted diffuse light but prevented pattern vision. Except when eating or at toilet, they wore cotton gloves and cardboard cuffs . . . in order to limit tactile perceptions. (p. 8)

The subjects stayed from 2 to 3 days. Twenty-five of the 29 subjects reported hallucinations, which usually were initially simple and became progressively more complex over time. Three of the subjects believed their visions to be real:

> One man thought that he saw things coming at him and showed head withdrawal quite consistently when this happened; a second was convinced that we were projecting pictures on his goggles by some sort of movie camera; a third felt that someone else was in the cubicle with him. (p. 17)

Merely monotonous environments, as in long-distance driving or flying, are now thought to be capable of generating symptoms. The following excerpt is taken from a series on psychiatric symptoms in military aviation:

> A pilot was flying a bomber at 40,000 feet and had been continuing straight and level for about an hour. There was a haze over the ground that prevented a proper view and rendered the horizon indistinct. The other member of the crew was sitting in a separate place out of the pilot's view, and the two men did not talk to each other. Suddenly the pilot felt detached from his surroundings and then had the strong impression that the aircraft had one wing down and was turning. Without consulting his instruments he corrected the attitude, but

the aircraft went to a spiral dive because it had in fact been flying straight and level. The pilot was very lucky to recover from the spiral dive, and when he landed the airframe was found to be distorted [from the stress caused by the dive].

On examining the pilot, no psychiatric abnormality was found. . . . As the man had no wish to give up flying and was in fact physically and mentally fit, he was offered an explanation of the phenomenon and was reassured. He returned to flying duties. (A. M. H. Bennett 1961, p. 166)

In this case, the symptoms (depersonalization and spatial disorientation), occurring as they did in a real-life situation, could easily have resulted in a fatal accident. In laboratory studies of model psychoses, the consequences are usually easily controlled. Particularly relevant to this discussion is the role of reassurance of the subject by the experimenter, after the experiment is over.

In all of the laboratory studies (as in this last case as well), the persons who have had "psychotic" experiences are reassured; they are told, for example, that the experiences they had were solely due to the situation that they were placed in, and that anyone else placed in such a situation would experience similar sensations. In other words, the implications of the rule-breaking for the rule-breaker's social status and self-conception are "normalized." Suppose, however, for purposes of argument, that a diabolical experiment was performed in which subjects, after having exhibited the psychotic symptoms under stress, were "labeled." That is, they were told that the symptoms were not a normal reaction, but a reliable indication of deep-seated psychological disorder in their personality. Suppose, in fact, that such labeling were continued in their ordinary lives. Would such a labeling process stabilize rule-breaking that would have otherwise been transitory? This question is considered under Proposition 3, following, and in Chapter 5.

Returning to the consideration of origins, rule-breaking finally can be seen as a volitional act of innovation or rebellion. Two examples from art history illustrate the deliberate breaking of residual rules. It is reported that the early reactions of the critics and the public to the paintings of the French impressionists were ones of disbelief and dismay; the colors, particularly, were thought to be so unreal as to be evidence of madness. It is ironic that in the ensuing struggle, the Impressionists and their followers effected some changes in the color norms of the public. Today, we accept the colors of the Impressionists without a second glance.

The Dada movement provides an example of an art movement deliberately conceived to violate, and thereby reject, existing standards of taste and value. The jewel-encrusted book of Dada, which was to contain the greatest treasures of contemporary civilization, was found to be filled with toilet paper, grass, and similar materials. A typical objet d'art produced by Dadaism was a fur-lined teacup. A climactic event in the movement was the Dada Exposition given at the Berlin Opera House. All of the celebrities of the German art world and dignitaries of the Weimar Republic were invited to attend the opening night. The first item of the evening was a poetry-reading contest, in which there were fourteen contestants. Since the fourteen read their poems simultaneously, the evening soon ended in a riot.

The examples of residual rule-breaking given here are not presented as scientifically impeccable instances of this type of behavior. There are many problems connected with reliability in these areas, particularly with the material on behavior resulting from drug ingestion and sleep and sensory deprivation. Much of this material is simply clinical or autobiographical impressions of single, isolated instances. In the studies that have been conducted, insufficient attention is usually paid to research design, systematic techniques of data collection, and devices to guard against experimenter or subject bias.

Of the many questions of a more general nature that are posed by these examples, one of the more interesting is, Are the "model psychoses" produced by drugs or food, sleep, or sensory deprivation actually identical to "natural" psychoses or, on the other hand, are the similarities only superficial, masking fundamental differences between the laboratory and the natural rule-breaking? The opinions of researchers are split on this issue. Many investigators state that model and real psychoses are basically the same. According to a report in the autobiographical, clinical, and experimental accounts of sensory deprivation, Bleuler's cardinal symptoms of schizophrenia frequently appear: disturbances of associations, disharmony of affect, autism, ambivalence, disruption of secondary thought processes accompanied by regression to primary processes, impairment of reality-testing capacity, distortion of body image, depersonalization, delusions, and hallucinations (Rosenzweig 1959, p. 326). Other researchers, however, insist that there are fundamental differences between experimental and genuine psychoses.

The controversy over model psychoses provides evidence of a basic difficulty in the scientific study of mental disorder. Although there is an enormous literature on the description of psychiatric symptoms, at this writing scientifically respectable descriptions of the major psychiatric symptoms, that is to say, descriptions that have been shown to be precise, reliable, and valid, do not exist (Scott 1958, pp. 29–45). It is not only that studies that demonstrate the precision, reliability, and validity of measures of symptomatic behavior have not been made, but that the very basis of such studies, operational definitions of psychiatric symptoms, have yet to be formulated. In physical medicine, there are instruments that yield easily verified, repeatable measures of disease symptoms; the thermometer used in detecting the presence of fever is an obvious example. The analogous instruments in psychiatric medicine, questionnaires, behavior rating scales, etc., which yield verifiable measures of the presence of some symptom pattern (e.g., paranoid ideation), have yet to be found, tested, and agreed upon.

In the absence of scientifically acceptable evidence, we can only rely on our own assessment of the evidence in conjunction with our appraisal of the conflicting opinions of the psychiatric investigators. In this case, there is at present no conclusive answer, but the weight of evidence seems to be that there is some likelihood that the model psychoses are not basically dissimilar to ordinary psychoses. Therefore, it appears that the first proposition, that there are many diverse sources of residual rule-breaking, is supported by available knowledge.

PREVALENCE

The second proposition concerns the prevalence of residual rule-breaking in entire and ostensibly normal populations. This prevalence is roughly analogous to what medical epidemiologists call the "total" or "true" prevalence of mental symptoms.

Proposition 2: *Relative to the rate of treated mental illness, the rate of unrecorded residual rule-breaking is extremely high.*

There is evidence that gross violations of rules are often not noticed or, if noticed, are rationalized as eccentricity. Apparently, many persons who are extremely withdrawn or who "fly off the handle" for extended periods of time, who imagine fantastic events, or who hear voices or see visions, are not labeled as insane either by themselves or others.[2] Their rule-breaking, rather, is unrecognized, ignored, or rationalized. This pattern of inattention and rationalization is called "normalization."[3]

In addition to the kind of evidence just cited, there are a number of epidemiological studies of total prevalence. There are numerous problems in interpreting the results of these studies; the major difficulty is that the definition of mental disorder is different in each study, as are the methods used to screen cases. These studies represent, however, the best available information and can be used to estimate total prevalence.

A convenient summary of findings is presented in Plunkett and Gordon (1960). These authors compare the methods and populations used in 11 field studies and list rates of total prevalence as 1.7, 3.6, 4.5, 4.7, 5.3, 6.1, 10.9, 13.8, 23.2, 23.3, and 33.3%.

Since the Plunkett and Gordon review was published, two elaborate studies of symptom prevalence have appeared, one in Manhattan, the other in Nova Scotia (Srole et al. 1962; Leighton et al. 1963). In the Midtown Manhattan study, it is reported that 80% of the sample currently had at least one psychiatric symptom. Probably more comparable to the earlier studies is their rating of "impaired because of psychiatric illness," which was applied to

23.4% of the population. In the Stirling County, Nova Scotia, studies, the estimate of current prevalence is 57%, with 20% classified as "psychiatric disorder with significant impairment."

How do these total rates compare with the rates of treated mental disorder? One of the studies cited by Plunkett and Gordon, the Baltimore study reported by Pasamanick (1963, pp. 151–155), is useful in this regard since it includes both treated and untreated rates. As compared with the untreated rate of 10.9%, the rate of treatment in state, VA, and private hospitals of Baltimore residents was 0.5% (ibid., p. 153). That is, for every mental patient there were approximately 20 untreated persons located by the survey. It is possible that the treated rate is too low, however, since patients treated by private physicians were not included. Judging from another study, the New Haven, Connecticut, study of treated prevalence, the number of patients treated in private practice is small in comparison with those hospitalized: over 70% of the patients located in that study were hospitalized even though extensive case-finding techniques were employed. The overall treated prevalence in the New Haven study was reported as 0.8%, a figure that is in good agreement with my estimate of 0.7% for the Baltimore study (Hollingshead and Redlich 1958, p. 199). If we accept 0.8% as an estimate of the upper limit of treated prevalence for the Pasamanick study, the ratio of treated to untreated patients is 1:14. That is, for every patient we should expect to find 14 untreated cases in the community.

One interpretation of this finding is that the untreated patients in the community represent those with less severe disorders, while patients with severe impairments all fall into the treated group. Some of the findings in the Pasamanick study point in this direction. Of the untreated patients, about half are classified as psychoneurotic. Of the psychoneurotics, in turn, about half again are classified as suffering from minimal impairment. At least a fourth of the untreated group, then, involved very mild disorders (Pasamanick 1963, pp. 153–154).

The evidence from the group diagnosed as psychotic does not support this interpretation, however. Almost all of the persons diagnosed as psychotic were judged to have severe impairment, yet half of the diagnoses of psychosis occurred in the untreated group. In other words, according to this study, there were as many untreated as treated cases of psychoses (ibid.).

In the Manhattan study, a direct comparison by age group was made between the most deviant group (those classified as "incapacitated") and persons actually receiving psychiatric treatment. The results for the groups of younger age (20–40 years) is similar to that in the Pasamanick study: Treated prevalence is roughly 0.6%, and the proportion classified as "incapacitated" is about 1.5%. In the older age group, however, the ratio of treated to treatable changes abruptly. The treated prevalence is about 0.5%, but 4% are designated as "incapacitated" in the population. In the older group, therefore, the ratio of treatable to treated (Srole et al. 1962) is about 8:1.

Once again, because of lack of complete comparability between studies, conflicting results, and inadequate research designs, the evidence regarding prevalence is not conclusive. The existing weight of evidence appears, however, very strongly to support Proposition 2.

THE DURATION AND CONSEQUENCES OF RESIDUAL RULE-BREAKING

In most epidemiological research, it is frequently assumed that treated prevalence is an excellent index of total prevalence. The community studies previously discussed, however, suggest that the majority of cases of "mental illness" never receive medical attention. This finding has great significance for a crucial question about residual deviance: given a typical instance of residual rule-breaking, what is its expected course and consequences? Or, to put the same question in medical language, what is the prognosis for a case in which psychiatric signs and symptoms are evident?

The usual working hypothesis for physicians confronted with a sign or symptom is that of progressive development as the inner logic of disease unfolds. The medical framework thus leads one to expect that unless medical intervention occurs, the signs and symptoms of disease are usually harbingers of further, and more serious, consequences for the individual showing the symptoms. This is not to say, of course, that physicians think of all symptoms as being parts of a progressive disease pattern; witness the concept of the "benign" condition. The point is that the imagery that the medical model calls up tends to predispose the physician toward expecting that symptoms are but initial signs of further illness.

The finding that the great majority of persons displaying psychiatric symptoms go untreated leads to the third proposition.

Proposition 3: *Most residual rule-breaking is normalized and is of transitory significance.*

The enormously high rates of total prevalence suggest that most residual rule-breaking is unrecognized or rationalized away. For this type of rule-breaking, which is amorphous and uncrystallized, Lemert used the term "primary deviation" (Lemert 1951, Chapter 4). Balint (1957) describes similar behavior as "the unorganized phase of illness" (p. 18). Although Balint assumes that patients in this phase ultimately "settle down" to an "organized illness," other outcomes are possible. A person in this stage may "organize" his deviance in other than illness terms (e.g., as eccentricity or genius), or the rule-breaking may terminate when situational stress is removed.

The experience of battlefield psychiatrists can be interpreted to support the hypothesis that residual rule-breaking is usually transitory. Glass (1953) reports that combat neurosis is often self-terminating if the soldier is kept with his unit and given only the most superficial medical attention.[4] Descriptions of child behavior can be interpreted in the same way. According to these reports, most children go through periods in which at least several of the following kinds of rule-breaking may occur: temper tantrums, head banging, scratching, pinching, biting, fantasy playmates or pets, illusory physical complaints, and fears of sounds, shapes, colors, persons, animals, darkness, weather, ghosts, and so on (Ilg and Ames 1960, pp. 138–188). In the vast majority of instances, however, these behavior patterns do not become stable.

There are, of course, conditions that do fit the model of a progressively unfolding disease. In the case of a patient exhibiting psychiatric symptoms because of general paresis, the early signs and symptoms appear to be good, though not perfect indicators of later more serious deterioration of both physical health and social behavior. Conditions that have been demonstrated to be of this type are relatively rare, however. Paresis, which was once a major category of mental disease, accounts today for only a very minor proportion of mental patients under treatment. Proposition 3 would appear to fit the great majority of mental patients, in whom external stress such as family conflict, fatigue, drugs, and similar factors are often encountered.

Of the first three propositions, the last is both the most crucial for the theory as a whole and the least well supported by existing evidence. It is not a matter of there being great amounts of negative evidence, showing that psychiatric symptoms are reliable indicators of subsequent disease, but that there is little evidence of any kind concerning development of symptoms over time. There are a number of analogies in the history of physical medicine, however, that are suggestive. For example, until the late 1940s, histoplasmosis was thought to be a rare tropical disease with a uniformly fatal outcome (Schwartz and Baum 1957). But it was later discovered that it is widely prevalent and with fatal outcome or even impairment extremely unusual. It is conceivable that most "mental illnesses" may prove to follow the same pattern when adequate longitudinal studies of cases in normal populations have been made.

If residual rule-breaking is highly prevalent among ostensibly "normal" persons and is usually transitory, as suggested by the last two propositions, what accounts for the small percentage of residual rule-breakers who go on to deviant careers? To put the question another way, under what conditions is residual rule-breaking stabilized? The conventional hypothesis is that the answer lies in the rule-breaker himself. The hypothesis suggested here is that an important factor (but not the only factor) in the stabilization of residual

rule-breaking is the societal reaction. Residual rule-breaking may be stabilized if it is defined to be evidence of mental illness and/or the rule-breaker
is placed in a deviant status and begins to play the role of the mentally ill. In
order to avoid the implication that mental disorder is merely role-playing and
pretense, it is necessary to discuss the social institution of insanity in the next
chapter.

NOTES

1. See Chapter 10 on the relationship between symptoms, context, and meaning.
2. See, for example, Clausen and Yarrow (1955), Hollingshead and Redlich (1958,
pp. 172–176), and E. Cumming and J. Cumming (1957, pp. 92–103).
3. The term *denial* is used in the same sense as in Cumming and Cumming (1957,
Chapter 7).
4. Cf. Kardiner and Spiegal (1947, Chapters 3–4).

5

The Social Institution of Insanity

Among psychiatrists, Szasz has been the most outspoken critic of the use of the medical model when applied to "mental illness." His criticism has taken the form that mental illness is a myth that serves functions that are largely nonmedical in nature:

> Our adversaries are not demons, witches, fate, or mental illness. We have no enemy whom we can fight, exorcise, or dispel by "cure." What we do have are problems in living—whether these be biologic, economic, political, or socio-psychological. . . . The field to which modern psychiatry addresses itself is vast, and I made no effort to encompass it all. My argument was limited to the proposition that mental illness is a myth, whose function it is to disguise and thus render more palatable the bitter pill of moral conflicts in human relations. (1960)

Szasz's formulations of the social, nonmedical functions that the idea of mental illness is made to serve are clear, cogent, and convincing. His conceptualization of the behavior that is symptomatic of "mental illness," however, is open to criticisms of a social-psychological nature.

In the "Myth of Mental Illness" (1960) Szasz proposes that mental disorder be viewed within the framework of "the game-playing model of human behavior" (pp. 113–118). He then describes hysteria, schizophrenia, and other mental disorders as the "impersonation" of sick persons by those whose "real"

69

problem concerns "problems of living." Although Szasz states that role-playing by mental patients may not be completely or even mostly voluntary, the implication is that mental disorder be viewed as a strategy chosen by the individual as a way of obtaining help from others. Thus, the term *imperson-ation* suggests calculated and deliberate shamming by the patient. Although he notes differences between behavior patterns of hysteria, malingering, and cheating, he suggests that these differences may be mostly a matter of whose point of view is taken in describing the behavior.

INDIVIDUAL AND INTERPERSONAL SYSTEMS IN ROLE-PLAYING

The present discussion also uses the role-playing model to analyze mental disorder but places more emphasis on the involuntary aspects of role-playing than Szasz, who tends to treat role-playing as an individual system of be-havior. In many social-psychological discussions, however, role-playing is considered as a part of a social system. The individual plays his role by ar-ticulating his behavior with the cues and actions of other persons involved in the transaction. The proper performance of a role is dependent on having a cooperative audience. The proposition may also be reversed: Having an au-dience that acts toward the individual in a uniform way may lead the actor to play the expected role even if he is not particularly interested in doing so. The "baby of the family" may come to find this role obnoxious, but the uni-form pattern of cues and actions that confronts him in the family may lock in with his own vocabulary of responses so that it is inconvenient and difficult for him not to play the part expected of him. To the degree that alternative roles are closed off, the proffered role may come to be the only way the in-dividual can cope with the situation.

One of Szasz's very apt formulations touches upon the social-systemic as-pects of role-playing. Szasz (1960) draws an analogy between the role of the mentally ill and the "type-casting" of actors.[1] Some actors get a reputation for playing one type of role, and find it difficult to obtain other roles. Although they may be displeased, they may also come to incorporate aspects of the typecast role into their self-conceptions and ultimately into their behavior. Findings in several social-psychological studies (Blau 1956; Benjamins 1950; Ellis 1945; Lieberman 1956) suggest that an individual's role behavior may be shaped by the kinds of "deference" that he regularly receives from others.[2]

One aspect of the voluntariness of role-playing is the extent to which the actor believes in the part he is playing. Although a role may be played cyni-cally, with no belief, or completely sincerely, with wholehearted belief, many roles are played on the basis of an intricate mixture of belief and disbelief. During the course of a study of a large public mental hospital, several pa-tients told the author in confidence about their cynical use of their symptoms—

to frighten new personnel, to escape from unpleasant work details, and so on. Yet, at other times, these same patients appear to have been sincere in their symptomatic behavior. Apparently, it was sometimes difficult for them to tell whether they were playing the role or the role was playing them. Certain types of symptomatology are quite interesting in this connection. In cases of patients simulating previous psychotic states and in the behavior pattern known to psychiatrists as the Ganser syndrome, it is apparently almost impossible for the observer to separate feigning of symptoms from involuntary acts with any degree of certainty.

The following case history excerpt from Sadow and Suslick (1961) will illustrate what psychiatrists have called simulation of a previous psychotic state:

A 32-year-old white man, an engineer, was readmitted to the hospital because of the recurrence of psychotic behavior. He had been hospitalized twice previously. The first time he had had electroshock treatment and had a remission for 4 years. One of us . . . saw him during his second hospitalization. At that time he was severely regressed, hallucinating freely, had magical and delusional behavior and many ideas of a messianic nature. He made a good functional recovery after several months of intensive psychotherapy by his private psychiatrist, supplemented with insulin coma treatment. Several years later he had a recurrence of symptoms and, because of my acquaintance with him during the previous hospitalization, he was referred by his previous therapist. On admission his behavior was bizarre enough to warrant sending him to the disturbed unit. There he immediately took over the unit claiming seniority rights because of his previous stay. When seen he was jovially patronizing, referred to his voices in a smiling manner and interspersed the interview with vague magical inferences of seemingly great significance. He continually made a particular gesture, that of a clock with the hands at the 6 o'clock position. This gesture had been the subject of much inquiry and work on his previous admission. As a result of the prior contact, it was possible to be more direct and inquiring with him than if he had been a new patient. At this point he gave no indications as to the precipitating stimulus of disruptive conflict. During some bantering in which he referred to his current hospitalization as a vacation, or a return of the old grad to his Alma Mater, he was told that this might prove to be an expensive class reunion. (This was in reference to one of his ostensible reasons for discontinuing psychotherapy following his previous disorder, namely, that treatment was too costly.) With almost dramatic swiftness following this remark, his bizarre behavior stopped and became quite depressed although still communicative. The following day it was possible to transfer him to a less controlled unit and he described in a completely coherent fashion with intense but appropriate emotion that he was extremely angry with his wife for nagging and belittling him. He was afraid he would not be able to control himself and felt that if he were sick like the last time he could avoid a feared outburst of physical violence by being hospitalized. In a few days he was able to recognize that much of the rage at his wife was directed at her current pregnancy. Although a moderate depression persisted, there was no recurrence of the bizarre behavior or the apparent hallucinations. He left the hospital after 3 weeks and returned directly to his job and home. (pp. 452–458)

What makes "simulation" particularly relevant to a social-systemic theory of mental illness is that it is believed that such behavior is usually a defensive reaction to external stress: "[This condition] consists of varying degrees of conscious simulation of the previous psychotic state by and under the control of the patient's ego when a subsequent situation of stress occurs" (Sadow and Suslick 1961, p. 452). This psychiatric definition closely parallels Lemert's (1951) sociological definition of "secondary deviation": "When a person begins to employ his deviant behavior or a role based upon it as a means of defense, attack, or adjustment to the overt and covert problems created by the consequent societal reaction, his deviation is secondary" (p. 76).

Moreover, it appears that such simulation can occur even where there has been no previous psychotic episode:

> A particularly striking example of this was seen in a young hospital record custodian who developed a complex of subjective symptoms highly suggestive of a frontal lobe brain tumor. Laboratory and physical tests short of air studies had revealed that her difficulties were of a conversion-like nature and were in part patterned after case histories that she had read with more diligence than called for by her job. (Sadow and Suslick 1961, p. 453)

Apparently, one can play the role of a mentally ill person without ever having actually experienced the role. Vicarious learning of imagery of the role of the mentally ill will be discussed shortly in the section following Proposition 5.

The Ganser syndrome appears to illustrate the intricate manner in which voluntary and involuntary elements intertwine in role-playing. This condition is referred to by psychiatrists as the "approximate answer" or *Vorbeireden* (talking past the point) syndrome:

> The patient is disoriented as to time and space and gives absurd answers to questions. Often he claims he does not know who he is, where he comes from, or where he is. When he is asked to do simple calculations, he makes obvious mistakes—for instance, giving 5 as the sum of 2 plus 2. When he is asked to identify objects, he gives the name of a related object. Upon being shown scissors, the patient may say they are knives; a picture of a dog may be identified as a cat, a yellow object may be called red, and so on. If he is asked what a hammer is used for, he may reply to cut wood. If he is shown a dime, he may state that it is a half-dollar and so on. If he is asked how many legs a horse has, he may reply, "Six."
> At times almost a game seems to go on between the examiner and the patient. The examiner asks questions that are almost silly in their simplicity, but

the patient succeeds in giving a sillier answer. And yet it seems that the patient understands the question, because the answer, although wrong, is related to the question. (Arieti, Silvano, and Meth 1959, p. 547)

In accordance with what has been said here about the social-systemic nature of role-playing, the difficulty in interpreting simulation of previous psychotic states, and the Ganser syndrome, is that the patient is just as confused by his own behavior as is the observer.

Some psychiatrists suspect that in schizophrenia there is a large element of behavior that is in the borderline zone between volitional and nonvolitional activity. Here are some excerpts from an autobiographical account of schizophrenia that stress the role-playing aspects:

> We schizophrenics say and do a lot of stuff that is unimportant, and then we mix important things in with all this to see if the doctor cares enough to see them and feel them.
>
> Patients laugh and posture when they see through the doctor who says he will help but really won't or can't. . . . They try to please the doctor but also confuse him so he won't go into anything important. When you find people who will really help, you don't need to distract them. You can act in a normal way.
>
> I can sense if the doctor not only wants to help but also can and will help . . .
>
> Patients kick and scream and fight when they aren't sure the doctor can see them. It's a most terrifying feeling to realize that the doctor can't understand what you feel and that he's just going ahead with his own ideas. I would start to feel that I was invisible or maybe not there at all. I had to make an uproar to see if the doctor would respond to me, not just his own ideas. (Hayward and Taylor 1956, p. 211)

Note that this patient has applied to herself a deviant label ("we schizophrenics"), and that her behavior fits Lemert's definition of secondary deviation; she appears to have used the deviant role as a means of adjustment.

This discussion suggests that a stable role performance may arise when the actor's role imagery locks in with the type of "deference" that he regularly receives. An extreme example of this process may be taken from anthropological and medical reports concerning the "dead role," as in deaths attributed to "bone-pointing." Death from bone-pointing appears to arise from the conjunction of two fundamental processes that characterize all social behavior. First, all individuals continually orient themselves by means of responses that are perceived in social interaction: The individual's identity and continuity of experience are dependent on these cues.

Generalizing from experimental findings, Blake and Mouton (1961) make this statement about the processes of conformity, resistance to influence, and conversion to a new role:

An individual requires a stable framework, including salient and firm reference points, in order to orient himself and to regulate his interactions with
others. This framework consists of external and internal anchorages available
to the individual whether he is aware of them or not. With an acceptable framework he can resist giving or accepting information that is inconsistent with the
framework or that requires him to relinquish it. In the absence of a stable framework he actively seeks to establish one through his own strivings by making use
of significant and relevant information provided within the context of interaction. By controlling the amount and kind of information available for orientation, he can be led to embrace conforming attitudes which are entirely foreign
to his earlier ways of thinking. (pp. 1–2)

Second, the individual has his own vocabulary of expectations, which may
in a particular situation either agree with or be in conflict with the sanctions
to which he is exposed. Entry into a role may be complete when this role is
part of the individual's expectations and when these expectations are reaffirmed in social interaction. In the following pages, this principle is applied
to the problem of the causation of mental disorder, through consideration of
the social institution of insanity.

LEARNING AND MAINTAINING ROLE IMAGERY

What are the beliefs and practices that constitute the social institution of insanity? And how do they figure in the development of mental disorder? Propositions 4 and 5 concerning beliefs about mental disorder in the general public
are now considered.

Proposition 4:   *Stereotyped imagery of mental disorder is learned in early
childhood.*

Although there are no substantiating studies in this area, scattered observations lead the author to conclude that children learn a considerable amount
of imagery concerning deviance very early, and that much of the imagery
comes from their peers rather than from adults. The literal meaning of *crazy,*
a term now used in a wide variety of contexts, is probably grasped by children during the first years of elementary school. Since adults are often vague
and evasive in their responses to questions in this area, an aura of mystery
surrounds it. In this socialization, the grossest stereotypes that are heir to
childhood fears (e.g., the bogeyman) survive. These conclusions are quite
speculative, of course, and need to be investigated systematically, possibly
with techniques similar to those used in studies of the early learning of racial
stereotypes.
    Here are some psychiatric observations on "playing crazy" in a group of
child patients (Cain 1964). This material indicates that the social stereotypes

are held by these children (ages 8–12) and play an active part in their cognition and behavior. It also fits the preceding discussion of role-playing and secondary deviation.

Equally prominent are their intense concerns about craziness, about the possibility that they themselves are crazy. . . . This concern seems to reflect the children's response to their own sporadic psychotic experience and behavior, a social awareness of how they appear to others, and perhaps in a sense an attempt to "explain" their own behavior. Undoubtedly, they are also reacting to teasing and name-calling by peers, and exasperated remarks by parents and teachers.

The child's concern about being crazy obtrudes in many different ways and places. Malcolm, in associating to his figure drawing, perseverates remarks about craziness: "He's a crazy person. He doesn't have a mind, just a nut. A nut, that's the way he is, he was born that way," "She's nuts, that's what people say about her—Hitler was nuts, wasn't he?" Gale enters her therapist's office obviously upset, abruptly refuses to talk of any worries, insists she's fine. Soon she tells of seeing a sign in the waiting room about lectures on emotionally disturbed children, and she cries out that she's not crazy. Bob accidentally cuts his finger in the occupational therapy shop. Badly shaking, he stares at the blood and yells, "My God, I'm going crazy." Another talks of only wanting Loony Tunes comics: "Loony Tunes," he snorts, "that's for me all right." Mark finds he has confused his craft shop days, is afraid that this means he's losing his mind. Many of the children use humor about or project these concerns . . . describing . . . other people as "crazy." They often focus their craziness, with or without past neurological exams and EEG's, upon their brain—"Got no brain. My brain is loose and swims around in my head. My brain and mind are no good, they get tired too quick," "Sometimes I get—it feels like explosions in my head. Something snaps up there. "

. . . A considerable component of the erratic behavior of these children has a conscious element—that is, they are "playing crazy." Much, though by no means all, of the playing crazy centers around their past experiences of and continual concerns about "being crazy." Their playing crazy takes many forms. It may be very quiet and subtle or blatant and obvious, identified as "pretend" by the child or exhaustively "defended" as crazy. Some of the varied forms are: "looking odd," staring off into space, or acting utterly confused; wild, primitive, disorganized rage like states; odd verbalizations, incoherences, mutterings; alleged hallucinations and delusions; the child's insistence that he is an animal, goblin, or other creature; or various grossly bizarre behaviors. Most of the children show many of these forms of playing crazy. Most of the children make clear—though by no means reliable—announcements that they have played crazy or intend to do so, or speak of "just pretending." The complex components of their playing crazy often become clear only after extended observation and therapeutic work.

At times, the child is quite consciously, deliberately, almost zestfully playing crazy—he is under no significant internal pressure, is completely in control, and at the end is most reassured. For if one can openly pretend to be crazy, how can one really be crazy? Not only current concerns but actual past incidents may thus be magically wiped away. Perhaps more frequently, playing crazy is used as other types of play are often used, namely, to achieve belated mastery of traumatic events, or anxiety-provoking internal states. . . .

At still other times—again not when under much pressure or anywhere near disintegration—the children pretend or toy with craziness, in a deliberate and controlled manner, as if they were almost experimenting with or testing attenuated psychotic experiences: the behavior somehow seems directed toward mastery of anticipated states rather than toward reduction of old anxieties. One feels that the child is saying, "What if such-and-such should happen . . . ?" or "What would it be like if . . . ?" It might well be labeled an "anti-surprise" measure, though clearly the previous psychotic states are not totally unrelated to this form of behavior, in which the child tentatively feels his way into feared future experiences of disintegration. Fenichel puts it well: " . . . a test action: repeating the overwhelming past and anticipating the possible future. 'Tensions are created,' . . . which might occur, but at a time and in a degree which is determined by the participant himself, and which is therefore under control."

At other times, when slipping toward or virtually in a psychotic state, the children may still attempt in a frenzied fashion to pretend to be crazy. Or perhaps more accurately, they pretend to be crazier than they are at that moment.

Sometimes the child keeps a sharp eye on his audience's reaction while producing a quite contrived, controlled production of craziness. He fretfully awaits a response as he asks an observer to define him. "Am I insane? Do you think I'm so insane, so out of control that I could really . . . behave this way?" Should the response be over-solicitous, he may be badly threatened by the possibility that he is what he fears and pretends to be. And he may angrily plead, as did Bart on such occasions, "I'm not that crazy!" (pp. 280–282; footnotes omitted)

Assuming that Proposition 4 is sound, what effect does early learning have on the shared conceptions of insanity held in the community? In early childhood, much fallacious material is learned that is later discarded when more adequate information replaces it. This question leads to Proposition 5.

Proposition 5:   *The stereotypes of insanity are continually reaffirmed, inadvertently, in ordinary social interaction.*

Although many adults become acquainted with medical concepts of mental illness, the traditional stereotypes are not discarded but continue to exist alongside the medical conceptions, because the stereotypes receive almost continual support from the mass media and in ordinary social discourse. In mental health education campaigns, televised lectures by psychiatrists and others, magazine articles and newspaper feature stories, medical discussions of mental illness occur from time to time. These types of discussions, however, seem to be far outnumbered by stereotypic references.

A study by Nunnally (1961) demonstrated that the portrait of mental illness in mass media is highly stereotyped. In a systematic and large-scale content analysis of television, radio, newspapers, and magazines, he found an image of mental disorder presented that was overwhelmingly stereotyped:

Media presentations emphasized the bizarre symptoms of the mentally ill. For example, information relating to factor I (the conception that mentally ill persons look and act different from "normal" people) was recorded 89 times. Of these, 88 affirm the factor, that is, indicated or suggested that people with mental health problems "look and act different": only one item denied factor 1. In television dramas, for example, the afflicted person often enters the scene staring glassy-eyed, with his mouth widely ajar, mumbling incoherent phrases or laughing uncontrollably. Even in what would be considered the milder disorders, neurotic phobias and obsessions, the afflicted person is presented as having bizarre facial expressions and actions (p. 74)

Of particular interest are the comparisons made between the imagery of mental disorder in the mass media, among mental health experts, and in the general public. In addition to the mass media analysis, data were collected from a group of psychiatrists and psychologists and from a sample drawn from the total population. The comparisons are summarized in Figure 5.1.

The solid line, representing the responses of the mental health experts, lies

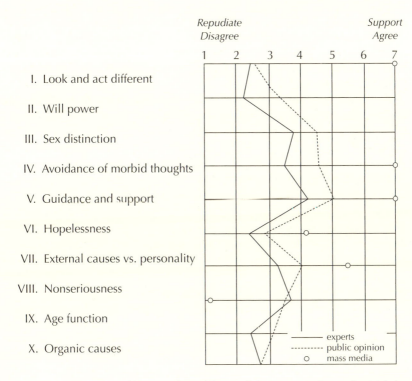
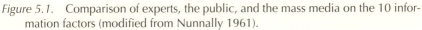

Figure 5.1. Comparison of experts, the public, and the mass media on the 10 information factors (modified from Nunnally 1961).

furthest to the left, in the direction of least stereotypy. The small circles—summarizing the findings in the study of the mass media—lie, for the most part, to the extreme right, the direction of greatest stereotypy. The broken line, indicating the findings of the sample survey in the public, lies between the mass media and the experts' profiles.

An interpretation of this finding is that the conceptions of mental disorder in the public are the resultant of cross-pressure: the opinions of experts, as expressed in mental health campaigns and "serious" mass media programming, pulling public opinion away from stereotypes, but with the more frequent and visible mass media productions reinforcing the traditional stereotypes.

Since Nunnally's sample of the mass media was taken during a single time period (one week of 1955), he makes no direct analysis of trends in time. However, he does present some direct evidence that is quite relevant to this discussion. He presents the number of television programs dealing with mental illness and subdivides them into documentary programs, which are presumably serious medical discussions, as contrasted with other programs; that is, features and films for each year during the period 1951–1958. His findings are presented in Table 5.1.

Once again, we see in the period 1957–1958 that the other features outnumber the serious programs by a ratio on the order of 100:1. Apparently, moreover, this disproportion was not decreasing, as many mental health workers believed, but actually increasing, as popular interest in mental disorder increases.

Although Nunnally's study represents a contribution to our knowledge of the imagery in the mass media and the general public, it is somewhat limited in terms of our present discussion, because the study deals only with direct references to mental illness and uses an incomplete set of categories for evaluating the references. The set of categories will be discussed first: Direct references are discussed shortly.

Table 5.1. Number of Television Programs Dealing with Mental Illness, 1951–1958*

	1951–53	1954	1955
Documentary programs	4	15	2
Other (features and films)	1	12	37
	1956	1957	1958
Documentary programs	2	1	1
Other (features and films)	122	169	72

* From Nunnally (1961).

The categories that are used in evaluating the content of the imagery of mental illness are of unequal interest; Category 1 ("Look and act different") and Category 6 ("hopelessness") are probably essential in understanding the mental illness imagery in the general public. There are other dimensions, however, that are not included in Nunnally's analysis, the most important of which are dangerousness, unpredictability, and negative evaluation. This can be made clear by referring to newspaper coverage of mental illness.

In newspapers it is a common practice to mention that a rapist or a murderer was once a mental patient. Here are several examples: Under the headline "Question Girl in Child Slaying," the story begins, "A 15-year-old girl with a history of mental illness is being questioned in connection with a kidnap-slaying of a 3-year-old boy." A similar story under the headline "Man Killed, Two Policemen Hurt in Hospital Fray" begins, "A former mental patient grabbed a policeman's revolver and began shooting at 15 persons in the receiving room of City Hospital No. 2 Thursday."

Often acts of violence will be connected with mental illness on the basis of little or no evidence. For instance, under the headline "Milwaukee Man Goes Berserk, Shoots Officer," the story describes the events and then quotes a police captain who said, "He may be a mental case." In another story, under the headline, "Texas Dad Kills Self, Four Children, Daughter Says," the last sentence of the story is "One report said Kinsey [the killer] was once a mental patient." In most large newspapers, there apparently is at least one such story in every issue.

Even if the coverage of these acts of violence were highly accurate, it would still give the reader a misleading impression, because negative information is seldom offset by positive reports. An item like the following is almost inconceivable: "Mrs. Ralph Jones, an ex–mental patient, was elected president of the Fairview Home and Garden Society at their meeting last Thursday."

Because of highly biased reporting, the reader is free to make the unwarranted inference that murder and rape and other acts of violence occur more frequently among former mental patients than among the population at large. Actually, it has been demonstrated that the incidence of crimes of violence (or of any crime) is much lower among former mental patients than in the general population.[3] Yet, because of newspaper practice, this is not the picture presented to the public. Newspapers have established an ineluctable relationship between mental illness and violence. Perhaps as importantly, this connection also signifies the incurability of mental disorder; that is, it connects former mental patients with violent and unpredictable acts.

It seems paradoxical that progress in communication techniques has created a situation in which the stereotyping process is probably growing stronger. Newspapers now use teletype releases from the press associations; and since these associations report incidents of crime and violence involving mental patients from the entire nation, the sampling bias in the picture presented to the public is enormous.

There are approximately 300,000 adults confined to mental hospitals in the United States on any one day, and an even larger group of former mental patients. The newspaper practice of daily reporting the violent acts of some patient or former patient and, at the same time, seldom indicating the size of the vast group of nonviolent patients is grossly misleading. Inadvertently, newspapers use selective reporting of the same type that is found in the most blatantly false advertisements and propaganda to continually "prove" that mental patients are unpredictably violent.

The impact of selective reportage is great because it confirms the public's stereotypes of insanity. Even if the newspaper were to explain the bias in these stories, the problem would not be eliminated. The vivid portrayal of a single case of human violence has more emotional impact on the reader than the statistics that indicate the true actuarial risks from mental patients as a class.

The average person's reaction to the fact that the probability of the kind of violence that the newspapers report occurring is about one in a million is usually that this is still a real risk that he will not accept. Yet this is roughly the risk of death he unthinkingly accepts in taking a cross-country trip in an airplane or automobile. One component of the stereotype of insanity is an unreasoned and unreasonable fear of mental patients that makes the public reluctant to take risks in this area of the same size as risks frequently encountered and accepted in the ordinary round of living.

Reaffirmation of the stereotype of insanity occurs not only in the mass media (see Figure 5.2) but indirectly in ordinary conversation: in jokes, in anecdotes, and even in conventional phrases. Such phrases as "Are you crazy?" "It would be a madhouse," "It's driving me out of my mind," "We were chatting like crazy," "He was running like mad," and literally hundreds of others occur frequently in informal conversations. In this usage, insanity itself is seldom the topic of conversation, and the discussants do not mean to refer to the topic of insanity and are usually unaware that they are doing so.

I have overheard mental patients, when talking among themselves, use these phrases unthinkingly. Even those mental health workers, such as psychiatrists, psychologists, and social workers, who are most interested in changing the concept of mental disorder often use these terms—sometimes jokingly but usually unthinkingly—in their informal discussions. These terms are so much a part of ordinary language that only the person who considers every word carefully can eliminate them from his speech. Through verbal usage, the stereotype of insanity is an inflexible part of the social structure.

The imagery that is implicit in these phrases should be discussed. When the phrase "running like mad" is used, the imagery that this conveys implicitly is movement of a wild and perhaps uncontrolled variety. The question

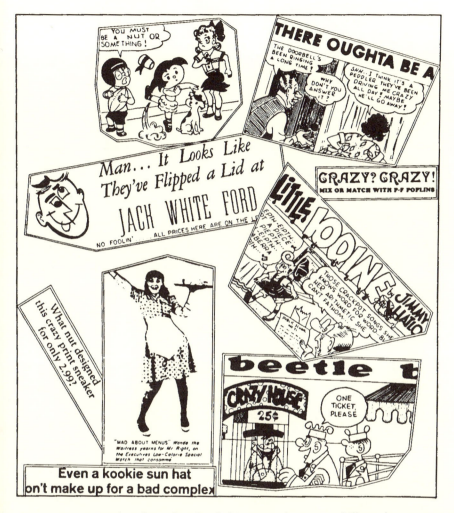

Figure 5.2. Examples of visual and verbal imagery about mental illness from newspapers and magazines.

"Are you out of your mind?" signifies a behavior of which the speaker disapproves. The frequently used term *crazy* often, although not always, implies subtle ridicule or stigma. These implications are there even when the person using the terms does not mean the words to convey this.

This inadvertent and incidental imagery is similar to that contained in racial and ethnic stereotypes. A speaker who uses the expression "to Jew someone down," may not necessarily be prejudiced against Jews (as in the rural South, where Jews are rare) but simply uses the phrase as a matter of convenience in order to convey his meaning; but to others the assumptions are unmistakable: the image of the Jew as a person who is scheming and overinterested in money for its own sake.

Again as in racial and ethnic stereotypes, imagery is sometimes conveyed through jokes and anecdotes. This example of the type of joke that one hears in informal conversation is taken from the *Reader's Digest*:

> A visitor to a mental hospital sees a patient who looks and acts like a normal person. He asks him why he is in the hospital. "Because I like potato pancakes," the patient replies. The visitor says, "That's nothing, I like potato pancakes myself." The patient turns to the visitor excitedly, "You do!" he replies, "Why don't you come to my room then, I have a whole trunkful!"

The implications that one may draw from this type of joke are fairly clear. Persons who are mentally ill, even when they do not seem to be, are basically different. This is one theme, among others, that recurs in reference to mental illness in ordinary conversation. This theme, together with the "looks and acts different" theme and the "incurable" theme, is probably part of a single larger pattern: These deviants (like other deviants) belong to a fundamentally different class of human beings or perhaps even a different species. This is a manifestation of outgrouping, the beliefs and actions that are based on the premise that one's enemies, strangers, or deviants, no matter how attractive or sympathetic they may seem to the unwary, are essentially different from and inferior to one's own kind.

Two racist jokes will provide an illustration of this genre:

> A black advertising executive is interviewed in his home, a luxurious apartment on the Hudson, on the television program "Person-to-Person." He is impeccably dressed, articulate, and speaks with the easy, cultivated accent of East Coast society. He says, "Good evening Ed." Ed Murrow says, "Good evening, Mr. Johnson." The executive introduces his family. Murrow says, "Before you take us on a tour of your home, could you tell our audience something about your working day?" Mr. Johnson says, "Certainly, Ed. On the typical weekday, my man comes around to pick me up about 9, and we get to the Avenue about 10. I have an accounts conference until 12, lunch and cocktails till 2. At 2 another accounts conference until 4, then I dictate letters until about 6. My man picks me up, I'm home by 7. As often as not, we have people over for dinner and drinks. They stay until 11 or 12, then I go out on the balcony, and jes look out ober de ribber."

A second, slightly less dated variant:

> As the plane taxis down the runway, the passengers of a jet hear over the intercom: "Good afternoon, ladies and gentlemen. I am your pilot." He delivers

the usual rundown on the flight, ending on this note: "I want you to know that I am the first black pilot hired by this airline. You are in good hands—I got my bachelor's at Harvard and my master's at MIT, graduating from both schools with honors. I have been through the same long rigorous training as all the white pilots, and received an award for being first in my class. I would like to tell you more, but right now I got to get this big motherfucker off the ground!"

These two jokes, and literally hundreds of other similar ones, all make exactly the same point: no matter how advanced the member of the outgroup might seem, fundamentally they are different.

To summarize this section: public stereotypes of mental illness are difficult to change because they receive continual although inadvertent support from the mass media and in ordinary conversation. In support of this proposition, evidence from several studies and the author's observations have been cited.

On the basis of this evidence, one would suspect that mental health campaigns that are based largely on disseminating information will be doomed to failure because of the overwhelming preponderance of stereotyped information and imagery to which the average person is exposed.

It is difficult to say at this time how the situation could be changed. In some media—television, for example—a definite attempt is made to "clean up" the references to mental illness. As Nunnally (1961) points out, however, these attempts are not particularly successful. While television has managed to eliminate virtually all the irreverent slang references to mental illness such as "goofball," "flipped," "nut," and "loony," there has been no attempt to change the visual imagery.

Why are these stereotypes resistant to change? One possible explanation is that they are functional for the current social order and tend to be integrated into the psychological makeup of all members of the society. Racial stereotypes may perform similar functions. In the southern part of the United States, for example, racial stereotypes are not fortuitous and isolated attitudes; rather, they are integral parts of the southerner's cognitive structure. The stereotype of the black fulfills the functions of a contrast conception, a reference point for making social comparisons and self-evaluations. One clue to the existence of contrast conceptions is a highly proliferated vocabulary of vernacular terms, such as exists in the South for referral to blacks. "Jig," "coon," "spade," "buck," and "jungle bunny" are only a few of an enormous number of such terms. In current vernacular, there is an equally large number of terms for referring to insanity, or going insane, for example: "out of one's mind," "losing one's mind," "the mind snapping," "out of one's head," "wrong in the head," "not right in the head" (or a gesture in which one moves the finger in a circle while pointing to one's head), "teched in the head," "cracked," "loony," "off one's rocker," "off the deep end," "nuts," "bughouse," "flipped," "psycho," "goofy," "ga-ga," "lose your marbles," "bats in the belfry" (or just "batty"), "screwy" or "screwball," "crazy," "deranged," "demented."

Judging from the frequency with which references to mental disorder appear in the mass media and in colloquial speech, the concept of mental disorder serves as a fundamental contrast conception in our society, functioning to preserve the current mores. The displacement of such a convenient concept is probably resisted for this reason. In some preliterate societies, the concept of spirit possession "explains" dreams, sickness, mental disorder, great success, untimely death, and many otherwise unexplainable phenomena. The average member of such a society has, therefore, a substantial psychological investment in the belief in spirit possession.

Similarly, in the United States, the average citizen resists changes in his concept of insanity—or, if he is in the middle class, his concept of mental disease—because these concepts are functional for maintaining his customary moral and cognitive world.

This section concludes with a discussion of a process that may relate stereotyping of the mentally ill to the social dynamics of mental illness: vicarious learning. The transmission of stereotyped imagery in the mass media and ordinary conversation may throw light on a question that has been hotly debated; whether the symptoms of mental disorder are inherent or learned. Although advocates of the learning point of view have pointed to instances where symptoms seemed to be learned (*folie a deux*, role models in the family), they have never been completely satisfied with this explanation, since it places so much emphasis on what seem to be infrequent occurrences.

The discussion here suggests that everyone in a society learns the symptoms of mental disorder vicariously through the imagery that is unintentionally conveyed in everyday life. This imagery tends to be tied to the vernacular of each language and culture; this association may be one reason why there are considerable variations in the symptoms of mental disorder that occur in different cultures. If, as suggested here, this imagery is available to the rule-breaker to structure and thus to "understand" his own experience, the quality of the societal reaction becomes extremely important in determining the duration and outcome of the initially amorphous and unstructured residual rule-breaking. The nature of the societal reaction is shown in the next section to be made up of alternative, indeed, mutually exclusive components: normalization or labeling.

NORMALIZATION AND LABELING

According to the analysis presented here, the traditional stereotypes of mental disorder are solidly entrenched in the population because they are learned early in childhood and are continuously reaffirmed in the mass media and in everyday conversation. How do these beliefs function in the processes leading to mental disorder? This question is considered first by referring to the earlier discussion of the societal reaction to residual rule-breaking.

It was stated that the usual reaction to residual rule-breaking is normalization and that in these cases most rule-breaking is transitory. The societal reaction to rule-breaking is not always normalization, however. In a small proportion of cases, the reaction goes the other way, exaggerating and at times distorting the extent and degree of the violation. This pattern or exaggeration, which we will call "labeling," has been noted by Garfinkel (1956) in his discussion of the "degradation" of officially recognized criminals. Goffman (1959) makes a similar point in his description of the "discrediting" of mental patients:

> [The patient's case record] is apparently not regularly used to record occasions when the patient showed capacity to cope honorably and effectively with difficult life situations. Nor is the case record typically used to provide a rough average of sampling of his past conduct. [Rather, it extracts] from his whole life course a list of those incidents that have or might have had "symptomatic" significance. . . . I think that most of the information gathered in case records is quite true, although it might seem also to be true that almost anyone's life course could yield up enough denigrating facts to provide grounds for the record's justification of commitment.

Apparently under some conditions, the societal reaction to rule-breaking is to seek out signs of abnormality in the deviant's history to show that he was always essentially a deviant.

The contrasting social reactions of normalization and labeling provides a means of answering two fundamental questions. First, if rule-breaking arises from diverse sources—physical, psychological, and situational—how does the uniformity of behavior that is associated with insanity develop? Second, if rule-breaking is usually transitory, how does it become stabilized in those patients who become chronically deviant? To summarize, what are the sources of uniformity and stability of deviant behavior?

In the approach taken here, the answer to this question is based on Propositions 4 and 5, that the role imagery of insanity is learned early in childhood and is reaffirmed in social interaction. In a crisis, when the deviance of an individual becomes a public issue, the traditional stereotype of insanity becomes the guiding imagery for action, both for those reacting to the deviant and, at times, for the deviant himself. When societal agents and persons around the deviant react to him uniformly in terms of the traditional stereotypes of insanity, his amorphous and unstructured rule-breaking tends to crystallize in conformity to these expectations, thus becoming similar to the behavior of other deviants classified as mentally ill, and stable over time. The process of becoming uniform and stable is completed when the traditional imagery becomes a part of the deviant's orientation for guiding his own behavior.

The idea that cultural stereotypes may stabilize residual rule-breaking and tend to produce uniformity in symptoms is supported by cross-cultural studies of mental disorder. Although some observers insist there are underlying similarities, many agree that there are enormous differences in the manifest symptoms of stable mental disorder between societies and great similarity within societies (Yap 1951).

These considerations suggest that the labeling process is a crucial contingency in most careers of residual deviance. Thus Glass (1953), who observed that neuropsychiatric causalities may not become mentally ill if they are kept with their unit, goes on to say that military experience with psychotherapy has been disappointing. Soldiers who are removed from their unit to a hospital, he states, often go on to become chronically impaired. That is, their deviance is stabilized by the labeling process, which is implicit in their removal and hospitalization. A similar interpretation can be made by comparing the observations of childhood disorders among Mexican-Americans with those of Anglo children. Childhood disorders such as *susto* (an illness believed to result from fright) sometimes have damaging outcomes in Mexican-American children (Saunders 1954, p. 142). Yet the deviant behavior involved is very similar to that which seems to have high incidence among Anglo children, with permanent impairment virtually never occurring. Apparently through cues from his elders, the Mexican-American child, behaving initially much like his Anglo counterpart, learns to enter the sick role, at times with serious consequences.[4]

ACCEPTANCE OF THE DEVIANT ROLE

From this point of view, most mental disorder can be considered to be a social role. This social role complements and reflects the status of the insane in the social structure. It is through the social processes that maintain the status of the insane that the varied rule-breaking from which mental disorder arises is made uniform and stable. The stabilization and uniformization of residual deviance are completed when the deviant accepts the role of the insane as the framework within which he organizes his own behavior. The three propositions stated below suggest some of the processes that cause the deviant to accept such a stigmatized role.

Proposition 6:   *Labeled deviants may be rewarded for playing the stereotyped deviant role.*

Ordinarily patients who display "insight" are rewarded by psychiatrists and other personnel. That is, patients who manage to find evidence of "their illness" in their past and present behavior, confirming the medical and societal diagnosis, receive benefits. This pattern of behavior is a special case of a more general pattern that has been called the "apostolic function" by Balint (1957), in which the physician and others inadvertently cause the patient to display symptoms of the illness the physician thinks the patient has. The apostolic function occurs in the context of bargaining between the patient and the doctor over what shall be decided to be the nature of the patient's illness:

> Some of the people who, for some reason or other, find it difficult to cope with problems of their lives resort to becoming ill. If the doctor has the opportunity of seeing them in the first phases of their being ill, i.e., before they settle down to a definite "organized" illness, he may observe that these patients, so to speak, offer or propose various illnesses, and that they have to go on offering new illnesses until between doctor and patient an agreement can be reached resulting in the acceptance by both of them of one of the illnesses as justified. (p. 18)

It is in this fluid situation that Balint believes the doctor influences the manifestations of illness:

> Apostolic mission or function means in the first place that every doctor has a vague, but almost unshakably firm, idea of how a patient ought to behave when ill. Although this idea is anything but explicit and concrete, it is immensely powerful, and influences, as we have found, practically every detail of the doctor's work with his patients. It was almost as if every doctor had revealed knowledge of what was right and what was wrong for patients to expect and to endure, and further, as if he had a sacred duty to convert to his faith all the ignorant and unbelieving among his patients. (p. 216)

Not only physicians but also other hospital personnel and even other patients reward the deviant for conforming to the stereotypes. Caudill, Redlich, Gilmore, and Brody (1952), who made observations of ward life in the guise of Caudill being a patient, reports various pressures from fellow patients. In the following excerpt, for example, there is the suggestion in the advice of the other patients that he should realize that he is a sick man:

> On the second day, following a conference with his therapist, the observer expressed resentment over not having going-out privileges to visit the library and work on his book—his compulsive concern over his inability to finish this task being (according to his simulated case history) one of the factors leading to his hospitalization. Immediately two patients, Mr. Hill and Mrs. Lewis, who were later to become his closest friends, told him he was being "defensive"; since his doctor did not wish him to do such work, it was probably better "to lay off it." Mr. Hill went on to say that one of his troubles when he first came to the hospital was thinking of things that he had to do or thought he had to do. He said that now he did not bother about anything. Mrs. Lewis said that at first

she had treated the hospital as a sort of hotel and had spent her therapeutic hours "charming" her doctor, but it had been pointed out to her by others that this was a mental hospital and that she should actively work with her doctor if she expected to get well. (p. 314–344)

In the California mental hospital in which the author conducted a study in 1959, a common theme in the discussions between patients on the admissions wards was the "recognition" of one's illness. This interchange, which took place during a ward meeting on a female admission ward, provides an extreme example:

New Patient:	I don't belong here. I don't like all these crazy people. When can I talk to the doctor? I've been here four days and I haven't seen the doctor. I'm not crazy.
Another Patient:	She says she's not crazy. (Laughter from patients.)
Another Patient:	Honey, what I'd like to know is, if you're not crazy, how did you get your ass in this hospital?
New Patient:	It's complicated, but I can explain. My husband and I . . .
First Patient:	That's what they all say. (General laughter.)

Thus there is considerable pressure on the patient to accept the role of the mentally ill as part of their self-conception.

Proposition 7: *Labeled deviants are punished when they attempt the return to conventional roles.*

The second process operative is the systematic blockage of entry to nondeviant roles once the label has been publicly applied.[5] Thus the former mental patient, although he is urged to rehabilitate himself in the community, usually finds himself discriminated against in seeking to return to his old status and on trying to find a new one in the occupational, marital, social, and other spheres.

Studies have shown that former mental patients, like ex-convicts, may find it difficult to find employment, even when their behavior and qualifications are unexceptionable. In an experimental study, Phillips (1963) has shown that the rejection of the mentally ill is largely a matter of stigmatization, rather than an evaluation of their behavior:

Despite the fact that the "normal" person is more an "ideal type" than a normal person, when he is described as having been in a mental hospital he is rejected more than psychotic individuals described as not seeking help or as seeing a clergyman, and more than a depressed-neurotic seeing a clergyman. Even when the normal person is described as [only] seeing a psychiatrist, he is rejected more than a simple schizophrenic who seeks no help, [and] more than a phobic-compulsive individual seeking no help or seeing a clergyman or physician. (pp. 963–973)

Propositions 6 and 7, taken together, suggest that to a degree the labeled deviant is rewarded for deviating and punished for attempting to conform.

Proposition 8:   *In the crisis occurring when a residual rule-breaker is publicly labeled, the deviant is highly suggestible and may accept the proffered role of the insane as the only alternative.*

When gross rule-breaking is publicly recognized and made an issue, the rule-breaker may be profoundly confused, anxious, and ashamed. In this crisis, it seems reasonable to assume that the rule-breaker will be suggestible to the cues that he gets from the reactions of others toward him.[6] But those around him are also in a crisis: the incomprehensible nature of the rule-breaking and the seeming need for immediate action lead them to take collective action against the rule-breaker on the basis of the attitude which all share—the traditional stereotypes of insanity. The rule-breaker is sensitive to the cues provided by these others and begins to think of himself in terms of the stereotyped role of insanity, which is part of his own role vocabulary also, since he—like those reacting to him—learned it early in childhood. In this situation, his behavior may begin to follow the pattern suggested by his own stereotypes and the reactions of others. That is, when a residual rule-breaker organizes his behavior within the framework of mental disorder, and when his organization is validated by others, particularly prestigeful others such as physicians, he is "hooked" and will proceed on a career of chronic deviance.

There is little direct evidence for the part played by role images in the development of mental illness, but there are various suggestions that it may be an important one. For example, Rogler and Hollingshead (1965), in their study of schizophrenia in Puerto Rico, give considerable emphasis to the role of the *loco* (lunatic) in the cases they studied. Comparing the 40 persons diagnosed as schizophrenic with the control group, they state:

> The role of the loco presents a problem to nearly all schizophrenic persons but to only a few who are free of the illness. Sick persons are extraordinarily defensive about the topic of the loco. Time and again, they state that they are not locos when no such question is being asked. When asked directly, only one sick person states that he is a loco; only one spouse of a sick person asserts this of his mate. The remaining persons in the sick group do not admit to locura. Rather, after a forceful denial, they add such phrases as: "Sometimes I act like one, but I am not one." "I may eventually become one, but I am not one now." "If I don't get help, I may become loco." "Perhaps I am on the road to becoming one." "Only at times do I act like a loco." (p. 221)

Although all but two of the 40 persons diagnosed as schizophrenic denied being loco in response to direct questions, the fact that they themselves raised the issue when the question was not asked suggests that the role image of the loco was being used in their own thought processes, regardless of their explicit denial. It is important for the reader to understand that the diagnosis of schizophrenia was made as part of the research process in this study and not necessarily officially in the community. The subjects were persons who had sought psychiatric help, and who were diagnosed as schizophrenic by a psychiatrist attached to the research group. From the point of view presented here, we may consider the "sick" (i.e., schizophrenic) group as persons who are experimenting with the role of the mentally ill.

Rogler and Hollingshead (1965) also found that the role image of the loco held by the "sick" group was not different from that held by the rest of the community:

> Schizophrenic persons are particularly vulnerable to being assigned the role of the loco. Consequently, we explored the possibility that the schizophrenic's portrayal of this role would be drawn in less harsh and more benign terms than that drawn by well people. This idea was erroneous! There is no tendency on the part of the schizophrenics to soften the portrait of the loco; sick and well persons describe him as violent, immoral, criminal, filthy, idiosyncratic, and worthless. Moreover, men and women do not differ in their conceptions of the loco. Their views are uniform and deep; perhaps they are fixed unalterably. (p. 218)

This finding is in accord with Propositions 4 and 5: if deviant role imagery is learned early and continually reaffirmed, a person's image of insanity would not likely be affected even when he himself runs the risk of being labeled. The role images are integral parts of the social structure and therefore not easily relinquished. Holding these relatively fixed images, the rule-breaker, like those around him, is susceptible to social suggestion in a crisis.

The role of suggestion is noted by Warner (1958) in his description of bone-pointing magic:

> The effect of [the suggestion of the entire community on the victim] is obviously drastic. An analogous situation in our society is hard to imagine. If all a man's near kin, his father, mother, brothers and sisters, wife, children, business associates, friends, and all the other members of the society, should suddenly withdraw themselves because of some dramatic circumstance, refusing to take any attitude but one of taboo   and then perform over him a sacred ceremony . . . the enormous suggestive power of this movement . . . of the community after it has had its attitudes [toward the victim] crystallized can be somewhat understood by ourselves. (p. 242)

If we substitute for black magic the taboo that usually accompanies mental disorder and consider a commitment proceeding or even mental hospital admission as a sacred ceremony, the similarity between Warner's description and the typical events in the development of mental disorder is considerable.

The last three propositions suggest that once a person has been placed in a deviant status, there are rewards for conforming to the deviant role and punishment for not conforming to the deviant role. This is not to imply, however, that the symptomatic behavior of persons occupying a deviant status is always a manifestation of conforming behavior. To explain this point, some discussion of the process of self-control in "normals" is necessary.

In a discussion of the process of self-control, Shibutani (1959, Chapter 6) notes that self-control is not automatic but is an intricate and delicately balanced process, sustainable only under propitious circumstances. He points out that fatigue, the reaction to narcotics, excessive excitement or tension (such as is generated in mobs), or a number of other conditions interfere with self-control; conversely, conditions that produce normal bodily states, and deliberative processes, such as symbolization and imaginative rehearsal before action, facilitate it.

One may argue that a crucially important aspect of imaginative rehearsal is the image of himself that the actor projects into his future action. Certainly in American society, the cultural image of the "normal" adult is that of a person endowed with self-control ("willpower," "backbone," or "strength of character"). For the person who sees himself as endowed with the trait of self-control, self-control is facilitated, since he can imagine himself enduring stress during his imaginative rehearsal and also while under actual stress.

For a person who has acquired an image of himself as lacking the ability to control his own actions, the process of self-control is likely to break down under stress. Such a person may feel that he has reached his "breaking-point" under circumstances that would be endured by a person with a "normal" self-conception. This is to say, a greater lack of self-control than can be explained by stress tends to appear in those roles for which the culture transmits imagery that emphasizes lack of self-control. In American society, such imagery is transmitted for the roles of the very young and very old, drunkards and drug addicts, gamblers, and the mentally ill.

Thus, the social role of the mentally ill has a different significance at different phases of residual deviance. When labeling first occurs, it merely gives a name to rule-breaking, which has other roots. When (and if) the rule-breaking becomes an issue and is not ignored or rationalized away, labeling may create a social type, a pattern of "symptomatic" behavior in conformity with the stereotyped expectations of others. Finally, to the extent that the deviant role becomes a part of the deviant's self-conception, his ability to control his own behavior may be impaired under stress, resulting in episodes of compulsive behavior.

The preceding eight hypotheses form the basis for the final causal hypothesis.

Proposition 9:   *Among residual rule-breakers, labeling is among the most important causes of careers of residual deviance.*

This proposition assumes that most residual rule-breaking, if it does not become the basis for entry into the sick role, will not lead to a deviant career.[7] The most usual case, according to the argument that has been advanced here, is that there will be few if any social consequences of residual rule-breaking. Occasionally, however, such rule-breaking may become the basis for major changes in the rule-breaker's social status, other than demotion to the status of a mental patient. The three excerpts that follow illustrate such shifts.

CASE 1:   Some of the Indian tribes of California accorded prestige principally to those who passed through certain trance experiences. Not all of these tribes believed that it was exclusively women who were so blessed, but among the Shasta this was the convention. Their shamans were women, and they were accorded the greatest prestige in the community. They were chosen because of their constitutional liability to trance and allied manifestations. One day the woman who was so destined, while she was about her usual work, fell suddenly to the ground. She had heard a voice speaking to her in tones of the greatest intensity. Turning, she had seen a man with drawn bow and arrow. He commanded her to sing on pain of being shot through the heart by his arrow, but under the stress of the experience she fell senseless. Her family gathered. She was lying rigidly, hardly breathing. They knew that for some time she had had dreams of a special character which indicated a shamanistic calling, dreams of escaping grizzly bears, falling off cliffs or trees, or of being surrounded by swarms of yellow-jackets. The community knew therefore what to expect. After a few hours the woman began to moan gently and to roll about upon the ground, trembling violently. She was supposed to be repeating the song which she had been told to sing and which during the trance had been taught her by the spirit itself, and immediately blood oozed from her mouth.

When the woman had come to herself after the first encounter with her spirit, she danced that night her first initiatory shaman's dance. For three nights she danced, holding herself by a rope that was swung from the ceiling. On the third night she had to receive in her body her power from the spirit. She was dancing, and as she felt the approach of the moment she called out, "He will shoot me, he will shoot me," Her friends stood close, for when she reeled in a kind of cataleptic seizure, they had to seize her before she fell or she would die. . . . From this time on she continued to validate her supernatural power by further cataleptic demonstrations, and she was called upon in great emergencies of life and death, for curing and for divination and for counsel. She became in other words, by this procedure a woman of great power and importance. (Benedict 1946, pp. 245–247)

CASE 2: [Samuel lived in the house of Eli, the priest. One night, as Samuel lay down, he heard a voice call his name] . . . and he answered, "Here am I." And he ran to Eli, and said, "Here am I; for thou callest me." And he said, "I called not; lie down again." And he went and lay down.

[Again Samuel heard his name called] . . . and Samuel arose and went to Eli, and said, "Here am I; for thou didst call me." And he answered, "I called not, my son; lie down again." [For the third time, Samuel heard his name called]. . . . And he arose and went to Eli, and said, "Here am I, for thou didst call me." And Eli perceived that the Lord had called the child.

Therefore Eli said unto Samuel, "Go, lie down: and it shall be, if He call thee, that you shall say, Speak, Lord, for thy servant heareth." So Samuel went and lay down in his place. And the Lord came, and stood, and called as at other times, "Samuel, Samuel." Then Samuel answered, "Speak, Lord, for thy servant heareth." [Samuel hears prophesied the downfall of the house of Eli]. . . . And all Israel from Dan even to Beersheba knew that Samuel was established to be a prophet of the Lord. (I Sam. 3:4–6, 8–10, 20)

CASE 3: INTERVIEWER: "How did you first come to believe that you had psychic powers, Mrs. Bendit:" ". . . during this particular period of my life, I was facing a number of personal problems that seemed overwhelming to me at the time. I was thoroughly depressed and confused, and I felt that the strain was getting progressively worse. I had been in this state for abut two weeks, when one Sunday morning, in church, I was shocked to see, up in the rafters of the ceiling of the church, a group of angels. I couldn't keep my eyes from the sight, although I noticed that no one else in the congregation was looking up. After this experience, I wandered around for several days, hardly knowing what to do with myself. One evening soon after, I went to a reception, hoping to take my mind from my troubles."

"I stayed pretty much to myself at the party, but I soon noticed, that across the room there was a woman who was watching me intently. She finally came over to me and introduced herself. She then explained clairvoyance to me at some length. I told her about my vision in the church, She explained that this experience was an example of my psychic powers. She said that she was a psychic, and that she could tell that I had the gift also. Although her explanation sounded strange to me, I felt somewhat relieved. In the ensuing weeks, I saw her often and we often had lengthy conversations. She introduced me into the group of clairvoyants and interested persons that she belonged to. . . . It was to this group that I first began to demonstrate my clairvoyance. . . . Several years after this I was able to arrange, with the help of my husband [her husband is a physician] an appearance before the Royal Academy of Medicine for a demonstration of clairvoyance."[8]

Cases 1 and 2 illustrate elevations in social status that are based on primary rule-breaking. Case 3 illustrates what may be called a lateral movement in status, since Mrs. Bendit has obviously become completely identified with her role as a clairvoyant.

The likelihood that residual rule-breaking in itself will not lead to labeling as a deviant draws attention to the central significance of the contingencies that influence the direction and intensity of the societal reaction. One of the urgent conceptual tasks for a sociological theory of deviant behavior is the development of a precise and widely applicable set of such contingencies. The classification that is offered here is only a crude first step in this direction.

Although a wide variety of contingencies lead to labeling, they can be simply classified in terms of the nature of the rule-breaking, the person who breaks the rules, and the community in which the rule-breaking occurs. Other things being equal, the severity of the societal reaction is a function of, first, the degree, amount, and visibility of the rule-breaking; second, the power of the rule-breaker and the social distance between him and the agents of social control; and finally, the tolerance level of the community and the availability in the culture of the community of alternative nondeviant roles.[9] Particularly crucial for future research is the importance of the first two contingencies (the amount and degree of rule-breaking), which are characteristics of the rule-breaker, relative to the remaining five contingencies, which are characteristics of the social system. To the extent that these five factors are found empirically to be independent determinants of labeling and denial, the status of the mental patient can be considered a partly ascribed rather than a completely achieved status. The dynamics of treated mental illness could then be profitably studied quite apart from the individual dynamics of mental disorder by focusing on social systemic contingencies.

A NOTE ON FEEDBACK IN DEVIANCE-AMPLIFYING SYSTEMS

It should be noted, however, that these contingencies are causal only because they become part of a dynamic system: the reciprocal and cumulative interrelation between the rule-breaker's behavior and the social reaction.[10] For example, the more the rule-breaker enters the role of the mentally ill, the more he is defined by others as mentally ill; but the more he is defined as mentally ill, the more fully he enters the role, and so on. This kind of vicious circle is quite characteristic of many different kinds of social and individual systems. It is very important to understand the part that social contingencies play in such a system, since the cause-effect relationship is not a simple one.

In the Rogler and Hollingshead (1965) study of schizophrenia in Puerto Rico, the authors drew attention to the dynamic interrelation between role entry and changes in the deviant's self-conception:

Although the sick person is deeply absorbed in his illness and yearns to speak about it, confidants are carefully selected. The illness is suppressed as a topic of conversation with friends and associates. Efforts are made to pretend that he is not a loco. He controls activities that exacerbate his loco-like behavior. These efforts are relatively futile, however, as the symptoms of the illness are strong and readily visible in the crowded social setting in which he lives. In point of fact, the sick person has begun to be viewed and treated as a loco. He withdraws from society out of fear that he will be stigmatized as a loco. In turn, the rejection by his friends and associates pushes him to withdraw. The stigma attached to this role is so strong that the withdrawal of the sick person from participation in all types of social groups appears to be a natural sequel to the condemnation he suffers. (pp. 241–242)

The process described in this passage can be interpreted as a vicious circle begun by stigmatization, withdrawal to avoid more stigma, stigmatization because of withdrawal or its effects, and so on around the circle.

The vicious circle effect occurs not only in the entrance to role-playing by the rule-breaker but in other parts of the system also. In order to see this more clearly, it is useful to represent the theory as a flowchart (Figure 5.3).[11]

This chart makes it clear that the theory of stable mental disorder discussed here is actually an assembly of system modules that interact. There is the module of residual rule-breaking; the contingency module, which filters out most of the rule-breakers through denial; the crisis module; the rule-breaker's self-conception module; the social control module, which operates such that the deviant tends to play the stereotyped deviant role; and finally, the compulsive behavior module. Each of these modules is a system in itself with its own contingencies. In the context of the larger theory, however, each is a subsystem, which under proper conditions, operates as part of the entire network.

The total system forms what Maruyama has called a "deviation-amplifying system," in which low-probability events are stabilized. In such a system, the simple causal laws in which similar conditions of deviance produce similar effects is not operative. Even more complicated models of contingent cause do not work, because it is necessary to specify the state of the entire system.

In cybernetic terms, what we have referred to as a vicious circle is called positive feedback, and it is apparent from the chart that there are a number of feedback loops in the system. The episodes of compulsive behavior interact with the earlier crisis, others' responses, and the deviant's self-conception subsystems, and the playing of the deviant role feeds back to the system of social control and the deviant's self-conception as well. Under proper conditions, deviation is not damped out by the action of the system, which is the usual situation in social systems, but is stabilized or even amplified.

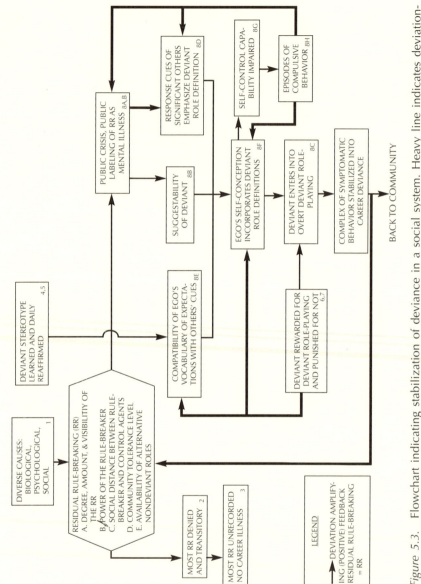

Figure 5.3. Flowchart indicating stabilization of deviance in a social system. Heavy line indicates deviation-amplifying (positive) feedback; RR: residual rule-breaking.

CONCLUSION

The discussion to this point has presented a sociological theory of the causation of stable mental disorder. Since the evidence advanced in support of the theory was scattered and fragmentary, it can only be suggested as a stimulus to further discussion and research. Among the areas pointed out for further investigation are field studies of the prevalence and duration of residual rule-breaking; investigations of stereotypes of mental disorder in children, the mass media, and adult conversations; studies of the rewarding of stereotyped deviation, of the blockage of return to conventional roles, and of the suggestibility of rule-breakers in crises. The final causal hypothesis suggests studies of the conditions under which normalization and labeling of residual rule-breaking occur. The variables that may effect the societal reaction concern the nature of the rule-breaking, the rule-breaker himself, and the community in which the rule-breaking occurs. Although many of the propositions suggested are largely unverified, they suggest avenues for investigating mental disorder different from those that are usually followed and the rudiments of a general theory of deviant behavior.

NOTES

1. For a discussion of type-casting, see Klapp (1962, pp. 5–8 passim).
2. For a review of experimental evidence, see Mann (1956). For an interesting demonstration of the interrelations between symptoms of patients on the same ward, see Kellam and Chassan (1962).
3. Brill and Malzberg (1950). See also Hastings (1958). Suicide is an important exception to these findings. The rate of suicide is reported in a number of studies as considerably higher among patients and ex-patients than among the rest of the population. Even though the relative rate is high, the absolute rate is still quite low. W. O. Hagstrom suggested this exception to me.
4. For a discussion, with many illustrative cases, of the process in which persons play the "dead role" and subsequently die, see Herbert (1961).
5. Lemert (1951) provides an extensive discussion of this process under the heading, "Limitation of Participation," pp. 434–440.
6. This proposition receives support from Erikson's (1957) observations.
7. Sociologically, an occupational career can be defined as "the sequence of movements from one position to another in an occupational system made by any individual who works in that system" (Becker 1963, p. 24). Similarly, a deviant career is the sequence of movements from one stigmatized position to another in the sector of the larger social system that functions to maintain social control. For example, the frequently cited progression of young men from probation through detention centers and reform schools to prison, with intervening times spent out of prison, may be considered as recurring deviant career. For his discussion of deviant careers, see Becker (1963, pp. 25–39).

8.   Interview on radio station KPFA, Berkeley, California, as recollected by the author.

9.   Cf. Lemert (1951, pp. 51–53, 55–68); Goffman (1959, pp. 134–135); Mechanic (1963). For a list of similar factors in the reaction to physical illness, see Koos (1954, pp. 30–38).

10.   For an explicit treatment of feedback, see Lemert (1962).

11.   W. Buckley suggested the use of this flowchart and provided help in interpreting the theory in cybernetic terms.

III

THE POWER OF THE PSYCHIATRIST

6

Decisions in Medicine[1]

The discussion to this point has concerned a theory of stable mental illness. In this chapter and the following chapter, our attention shifts from theory to practice. This chapter discusses a decision-making problem that psychiatry shares with general medicine. Members of professions such as law and medicine frequently are confronted with uncertainty in the course of their routine duties. In these circumstances, informal norms have developed for handling uncertainty so that paralyzing hesitation is avoided. These norms are based upon assumptions that some types of error are more to be avoided than others—assumptions so basic that they are usually taken for granted, are seldom discussed, and are therefore slow to change.

The purpose of this chapter is to describe one important norm for handling uncertainty in medical diagnosis, that judging a sick person well is more to be avoided than judging a well person sick, and to suggest some of the consequences of the application of this norm in medical practice. Apparently this norm, like many important cultural norms, "goes without saying" in the subculture of the medical profession; in form, however, it resembles any decision rule for guiding behavior under conditions of uncertainty. In the discussion that follows, decision rules in law, statistics, and medicine are compared in order to indicate the types of error that are thought to be the more important to avoid and the assumptions underlying this preference. On the basis of recent findings of the widespread distribution of elements of disease and deviance in normal populations, the assumption of a uniform relationship between disease signs and impairment is criticized. Finally, it is suggested that to the extent that physicians are guided by this medical decision rule, they too often place patients in the "sick role" who could otherwise have continued in their normal pursuits.

To the extent that physicians and the public are biased toward treatment, the "creation" of illness (i.e., the production of unnecessary impairment) may go hand in hand with the prevention and treatment of disease in modern medicine. The magnitude of the bias toward treatment in any single case may be quite small, since there are probably other medical decision rules ("When in doubt, delay your decision") that counteract the rule discussed here. Even a small bias, however, if it is relatively constant throughout Western society, can have effects of large magnitude. Since this argument is based largely on fragmentary evidence, it is intended merely to stimulate further discussion and research rather than to demonstrate the validity of a point of view. The discussion begins with the consideration of a decision rule in law.

In criminal trials in England and the United States, there is an explicit rule for arriving at decisions in the face of uncertainty: A man is innocent until proven guilty. The meaning of this rule is made clear by the English common-law definition of the phrase "proven guilty," which, according to tradition, is that the judge or jury must find the evidence of guilt compelling *beyond a reasonable doubt*. The basic legal rule for arriving at a decision in the face of uncertainty may be briefly stated: When in doubt, acquit. That is, the jury or judge must not be equally wary of erroneously convicting or acquitting: the error that is most important to avoid is to erroneously convict. This concept is expressed in the maxim, "Better a thousand guilty men go free, than one innocent man be convicted."

The reasons underlying this rule seem clear. It is assumed that in most cases a conviction will do irreversible harm to an individual by damaging his reputation in the eyes of his fellows. The individual is seen as weak and defenseless relative to society, and therefore in no position to sustain the consequences of an erroneous decision. An erroneous acquittal, on the other hand, damages society. If an individual who has actually committed a crime is not punished, he may commit the crime again, or more important, the deterrent effect of punishment for the violation of this crime may be diminished for others. Although these are serious outcomes, they are generally thought not to be so serious as the consequences of erroneous conviction for the innocent individual, since society is able to sustain an indefinite number of such errors without serious consequences. For these and perhaps other reasons, the decision rule to assume innocence exerts a powerful influence on legal proceedings.

TYPE 1 AND TYPE 2 ERRORS

Deciding on guilt or innocence is a special case of a problem to which statisticians have given considerable attention: the testing of hypotheses. Since most scientific work is done with samples, statisticians have developed techniques to guard against results that are due to chance sampling fluctuations. The problem, however, is that one may reject a finding that was actually correct as due to sampling fluctuations. There are, therefore, two kinds of errors: rejecting a hypothesis that is true and accepting one that is false. Usually the hypothesis is stated so that the former error (rejecting a hypothesis that is true) is the error that is thought to be the more important to avoid. This type of error is called an "error of the first kind," or a Type 1 error. The latter error (accepting a hypothesis that is false) is the less important error to avoid and is called an "error of the second kind," or a Type 2 error (Neyman 1950, pp. 265–266).

To guard against chance fluctuations in sampling, statisticians test the probability that findings could have arisen by chance. At some predetermined probability (called the "alpha level"), usually 0.05 or less, the possibility that the findings arose by chance is rejected. This level means that there are 5 chances in 100 that one will reject a hypothesis that is true. Although these 5 chances indicate a real risk of error, it is not common to set the level much lower (say 0.001) because this raises the probability of making an error of the second kind.

A similar dilemma faces the judge or jury in deciding whether to convict or acquit in the face of uncertainty. Particularly in the adversary system of law, where professional attorneys seek to advance their arguments and refute those of their opponents, there is often considerable uncertainty even as to the facts of the case, let alone intangibles like intent. The maxim, "Better a thousand guilty men go free, than one innocent man be convicted," would mean, if taken literally rather than as a rhetorical flourish, that the alpha level for legal decisions is set quite low.

Although the legal decision rule is not expressed in so precise a form as a statistical decision rule, it represents a very similar procedure for dealing with uncertainty. There is one respect, however, in which it is quite different. Statistical decision procedures are recognized by those who use them as mere conveniences, which can be varied according to the circumstances. The legal decision rule, in contrast, is an inflexible and binding moral rule, which carries with it the force of long sanction and tradition. The assumption of innocence is a part of the social institution of law in Western society; it is explicitly stated in legal codes and is accepted as legitimate by jurists and usually by the general populace with only occasional grumbling (e.g., a criminal is seen as "getting off" because of "legal technicalities").

DECISION RULES IN MEDICINE

Although the analogous rule for decisions in medicine is not so explicitly stated as the rule in law and probably is considerably less rigid, it would seem that there is such a rule in medicine, which is as imperative in its operation as its analog in law. Which error do physicians and the general public consider it most important to avoid: rejecting the hypothesis of illness when it is true, or accepting it when it is false? It seems fairly clear that the rule in medicine may be stated as: "When in doubt, continue to suspect illness." That is, for a physician to dismiss a patient when he is actually ill is a Type 1 error, and to retain a patient when he is not ill is a Type 2 error.

Most physicians learn early in their training that it is far more culpable to dismiss a sick patient than to retain a well one. This rule is so pervasive and fundamental that it goes unstated in textbooks on diagnosis. It is occasionally mentioned explicitly in other contexts, however. Neyman (1950), for example, in his discussion of X-ray screening for tuberculosis states:

> [If the patient is actually well, but the hypothesis that he is sick is accepted, a Type 2 error,] then the patient will suffer some unjustified anxiety and, perhaps, will be put to some unnecessary expense until further studies of his health will establish that any alarm about the state of his chest is unfounded. Also, the unjustified precautions ordered by the clinic may somewhat affect its reputation. On the other hand, should the hypothesis [of sickness] be true and yet the accepted hypothesis be [that he is well, a Type I error], then the patient will be in danger of losing the precious opportunity of treating the incipient disease in its beginning stages when the cure is not so difficult. Furthermore, the oversight by the clinic's specialist of the dangerous condition would affect the clinic's reputation even more than the unnecessary alarm. From this point of view, it appears that the error of rejecting the hypothesis [of sickness] when it is true is *far more important to* avoid than the error of accepting the hypothesis [of illness] when it is false. (p. 270; italics added)

Although this particular discussion pertains to tuberculosis, it is pertinent to many other diseases also. From casual conversations with physicians, the impression one gains is that this moral lesson is deeply ingrained in the physician's personal code.

It is not only physicians who feel this way, however. This rule is grounded both in legal proceedings and in popular sentiment. Although there is some sentiment against Type 2 errors (unnecessary surgery, for instance), it has nothing like the force and urgency of the sentiment against Type I errors. A physician who dismisses a patient who subsequently dies of a disease that should have been detected is subject not only to legal action for negligence and possible loss of license for incompetence, but also to moral condemnation from his colleagues and from his own conscience for his delinquency.

Nothing remotely resembling this amount of moral and legal suasion is brought to bear for committing a Type 2 error. Indeed, this error is sometimes seen as sound clinical practice, indicating a healthily conservative approach to medicine.

The discussion to this point suggests that physicians follow a decision rule that may be stated, "When in doubt, diagnose illness." If physicians are actually influenced by this rule, then studies of the validity of diagnosis should demonstrate the operation of the rule. That is, we should expect that objective studies of diagnostic errors should show that Type 1 and Type 2 errors do not occur with equal frequency, but in fact, that Type 2 errors far outnumber Type 1 errors. Unfortunately for our purposes, however, there are apparently only a few studies that provide the type of data that would adequately test the hypothesis. Although studies of the reliability of diagnosis abound (Garland 1959) showing that physicians disagree with each other in their diagnoses of the same patients, these studies do not report the validity of diagnosis or the types of error that are made, with the following exceptions.

We can infer that Type 2 errors outnumber Type 1 errors from Bakwin's (1945) study of physicians' judgments regarding the advisability of tonsillectomy for 1000 school children:

> Of these, some 611 had had their tonsils removed. The remaining 389 were then examined by other physicians, and 174 were selected for tonsillectomy. This left 215 children whose tonsils were apparently normal. Another group of doctors was put to work examining these 215 children, and 99 of them were adjudged in need of tonsillectomy. Still another group of doctors was then employed to examine the remaining children, and nearly one-half were recommended for operation. (pp. 691–697)

Almost half of each group of children were judged to be in need of the operation. Even assuming that a small proportion of children needing tonsillectomy were missed in each examination (Type 1 error), the number of Type 2 errors in this study far exceeded the number of Type 1 errors.

In the field of roentgenology, studies of diagnostic error are apparently more highly developed than in other areas of medicine. Garland (1959, p. 31) summarizes these findings, reporting that in a study of 14,867 films for tuberculosis signs, there were 1216 positive readings that turned out to be clinically negative (Type 2 error) and only 24 negative readings that turned out to be clinically active (Type 1 error)! This ratio (about 50:1) is apparently a fairly typical finding in roentgenographic studies. Since physicians are well aware of the provisional nature of radiological findings, this great discrepancy between the frequency of the types of error in film screening is not too alarming. On the other hand, it does provide objective evidence of the operation of the decision rule, "Better safe than sorry."

BASIC ASSUMPTIONS

The logic of this decision rule rests on two assumptions: First, disease is usually a determinate, inevitably unfolding process, which, if undetected and untreated, will grow to a point where it endangers the life or limb of the individual and, in the case of contagious diseases, the lives of others. This is not to say, of course, that physicians think of all diseases as determinate: Witness the concept of the "benign" condition. The point here is that the imagery of disease that the physician uses in attempting to reach a decision, his working hypothesis, *is usually* based on the deterministic model of disease. Second, medical diagnosis of illness, unlike legal judgment, is not an irreversible act that does untold damage to the status and reputation of the patient. A physician may search for illness for an indefinitely long time, causing inconvenience for the patient, perhaps, but in the typical case, doing the patient no irradicable harm. Obviously, again, physicians do not always make this assumption. A physician who suspects epilepsy in a truck driver knows full well that his patient will probably never drive a truck again if the diagnosis is made, and the physician will go to great lengths to avoid a Type 2 error in this situation. Similarly, if a physician suspects that a particular patient has hypochondriacal trends, the physician will lean in the direction of a Type 1 error in a situation of uncertainty. These and other similar situations are exceptions, however. The physician's *usual* working assumption is that medical observation and diagnosis, in itself, is neutral and innocuous relative to the dangers resulting from disease.[2]

In the light of these two assumptions, therefore, it is seen as far better for the physician to chance a Type 2 error than a Type I error. These two assumptions will be examined and criticized in the remainder of the chapter. The assumption that Type 2 errors are relatively harmless will be considered first.

In recent discussions, it is increasingly recognized that in one area of medicine, psychiatry, the assumption that medical diagnosis can cause no irreversible harm to the patient's status is dubious. Psychiatric treatment, in many segments of the population and for many occupations, raises a question about the person's social status. It could be argued that in making a medical diagnosis the psychiatrist comes very close to making a legal decision, with its ensuing consequences for the person's reputation. One may argue that the Type 2 error in psychiatry, of judging a well person sick, is at least as much to be avoided as the Type I error, of judging the sick person well. Yet the psychiatrist's moral orientation, since he is first and foremost a physician, is guided by the medical, rather than the legal, decision rule. The psychiatrist continues to be more willing to err on the conservative side, to diagnose as ill when the person is healthy, even though it is no longer clear that this error is any more desirable than its opposite.

There is a more fundamental question about this decision rule, however, which concerns both physical illness and mental disorder. This question primarily concerns the first assumption: that disease is a determinate process. It also implicates the second assumption: that medical treatment does not have irreversible effects.

In recent years, physicians and social scientists have reported finding disease signs and deviant behavior prevalent in normal, noninstitutionalized populations. It has been shown, for instance, that deviant acts, some of a serious nature, are widely admitted by persons in random samples of normal populations (Wallerstein and Wyle 1947; Porterfield 1946; Kinsey, Pomeroy, and Martin 1948). There is some evidence that suggests that grossly deviant, "psychotic" behavior has at least temporarily existed in relatively large proportions of a normal population (Plunkett and Gordon 1960; Clausen and Yarrow 1955). Finally, there is a growing body of evidence that many signs of physical disease are distributed quite widely in normal populations. A survey of simple high blood pressure indicated that the prevalence ranged from 11.4 to 37.2% in the various subgroups studied (Rautaharju, Korvonen, and Keys 1961).[3]

As stated in Chapter 4, physical defects and "psychiatric" deviancy exist in an uncrystallized form in large segments of the population. Lemert (1951) calls this type of behavior, which is often transitory, *primary deviation*. In his discussion of the doctor-patient relationship, Balint (1957) speaks of similar behavior as the "unorganized phase of illness" Balint seems to take for granted, however, that patients will eventually "settle down" to an "organized" illness. Yet it is possible that other outcomes may occur. A person in this stage may change jobs or wives instead, or merely continue in the primary deviation state indefinitely, without getting better or worse.

This discussion suggests that in order to estimate the probability that a person with a disease sign would become incapacitated because of the development of disease, investigations quite unlike existing studies would need to be conducted. These would be longitudinal studies in a random sample of a normal population, of outcomes in persons having signs of diseases in which no attempt was made to arrest the disease. It is true that there are a number of longitudinal studies in which the effects of treatment are compared with the effects of nontreatment. These studies, however, have always been conducted with clinical groups rather than with persons with disease signs who were located in field studies.[4] Even clinical trials appear to offer many difficulties, both from the ethical and scientific points of view (Hill 1960). These difficulties would be increased many times in controlled field trials, as would the problems that concern the amount of time and money necessary. Without such studies, nevertheless, the meaning of many common disease signs remains somewhat equivocal.

Given the relatively small amount of knowledge about the distributions and natural outcomes of many diseases, it is possible that our conceptions of the danger of disease are exaggerated. To mention again the dramatic example cited earlier, until the late 1940s, histoplasmosis was thought to be a rare tropical disease with a uniform fatal outcome. Recently, however, it was discovered that it is widely prevalent and with fatal outcome or impairment extremely rare (Schwartz and Baum 1957). It is conceivable that other diseases, such as some types of heart disease and mental disorder, may prove to be similar in character. Although no actuarial studies have been made that would yield the true probabilities of impairment, physicians usually set the Type 1 level quite high because they believe that the probability of impairment from making a Type 2 error is quite low. Let us now examine that assumption.

THE "SICK ROLE"

If, as has been argued here, much illness goes unattended without serious consequences, the assumption that medical diagnosis has no irreversible effects on the patients seems questionable.

> The patient's attitude to his illness is usually considerably changed during, and by, the series of physical examinations. These changes, which may profoundly influence the course of a chronic illness, are not taken seriously by the medical profession and, though occasionally mentioned, they have never been the subject of a proper scientific investigation. (Balint 1957, p. 43)

There are grounds for believing that persons who avail themselves of professional services are under considerable strain and tension (if the problem could have been easily solved, they would probably have used more informal means of handling it). Social-psychological principles indicate that persons under strain are highly suggestible, particularly to suggestions from a prestigious source, such as a physician.

It can be argued that the Type 2 error involves the danger of having a person enter the "sick role" (Parsons 1950) in circumstances where no serious result would ensue if the illness were unattended. Perhaps the combination of a physician determined to find disease *signs,* if they are to be found, and the suggestible patient, searching for subjective *symptoms* among the many amorphous and usually unattended bodily impulses, is often sufficient to uncarth a disease that changes the patient's status from that of well to sick and may also have effect on his familial and occupational status. [In Lemert's (1951) terms, the illness would be *secondary deviation* after the person has entered the sick role.]

There is a considerable body of evidence in the medical literature concerning the process in which the physician unnecessarily causes the patient to enter the sick role. Thus, in a discussion of "iatrogenic" (physician-induced) heart disease, this point is made:

> The physician, by calling attention to a murmur or some cardiovascular abnormality, even though functionally insignificant, may precipitate [symptoms of heart disease]. The experience of the work classification units of cardiac-in-industry programs, where patients with cardiovascular disease are evaluated as to work capacity, gives impressive evidence regarding the high incidence of such functional manifestations in persons with the diagnosis of cardiac lesion. (Warren and Wolter 1954, pp. 77–84)

Although there is a tendency in medicine to dismiss this process as due to quirks of particular patients (e.g., as malingering, hypochondriasis, or as "merely functional disease," that is, functional for the patient), causation probably lies not in the patient but in medical procedures. Most people, perhaps, if they actually have the disease signs and are told by an authority, the physician, that they are ill, will obligingly come up with appropriate symptoms. A case history will illustrate this process. Under the heading, "It may be well to let sleeping dogs lie," a physician recounts the following case:

> Here is a woman, aged 40 years, who is admitted with symptoms of congestive cardiac failure, valvular disease, mitral stenosis and auricular fibrillation. She tells us that she did not know that there was anything wrong with her heart and that she had had no symptoms up to 5 years ago when her chest was x-rayed in the course of a mass radiography examination for tuberculosis. She was not suspected and this was only done in the course of routine at the factory. Her lungs were pronounced clear but she was told that she had an enlarged heart and was advised to go to a hospital for investigation and treatment. From that time she began to suffer from symptoms—breathlessness on exertion—and has been in the hospital 4 or 5 times since. Now she is here with congestive heart failure. She cannot understand why, from the time that her enlarged heart was discovered, she began to get symptoms. (Gardiner-Hill 1958, p. 158)

What makes this kind of "role-taking" extremely important is that it can occur even when the diagnostic label is kept from the patient. By the way he is handled, the patient can usually infer the nature of the diagnosis, since in his uncertainty and anxiety he is extremely sensitive to subtleties in the physician's behavior. An example of this process (already cited in Chapter 4) is found in reports on treatment of battle fatigue. Speaking of psychiatric patients in the Sicilian campaign during World War II, a psychiatrist notes:

> Although patients were received at this hospital within 24 to 48 hours after their breakdown, a disappointing number, approximately 15 per cent, were salvaged for combat duty. . . . [A]ny therapy, including usual interview methods that

sought to uncover basic emotional conflicts or attempted to relate current behavior and symptoms with past personality patterns seemingly provided patients with logical reasons for their combat failure. The insights obtained by
even such mild depth therapy readily convinced the patient and often his therapist that the limit of combat endurance had been reached as proved by vulnerable personality traits. Patients were obligingly cooperative in supplying
details of their neurotic childhood, previous emotional difficulties, lack of ag-
gressiveness and other dependence traits. (Glass 1953)

Glass goes on to say that removal of the soldier from his unit for treatment
of any kind usually resulted in long-term neurosis. In contrast, if the soldier
were given only superficial psychiatric attention and *kept with his unit,* chronic
impairment was usually avoided. The implication is that removal from the
military unit and psychiatric treatment symbolizes to the soldier, behaviorally
rather than with verbal labels, the "fact" that he is a mental case.

The traditional way of interpreting these reactions of the soldiers, and
perhaps the civilian cases, is in terms of malingering or feigning illness. The
process of taking roles, however, as it is conceived of here, is not completely
or even largely voluntary. [For a sophisticated discussion of role-playing, see
Goffman (1959, pp. 17–21).] Vaguely defined impulses become "real" to the
participants when they are organized under any one of a number of more or
less interchangeable social roles. It can be argued that when a person is in a
confused and suggestible state, when he organizes his feelings and behavior
by using the sick role and when his choice of roles is validated by a physician
or others, he is "hooked" and will proceed on a career of chronic illness.[5]

IMPLICATIONS FOR RESEARCH

The hypothesis suggested by the preceding discussion is that physicians
and the public typically overvalue medical treatment relative to nontreatment
as a course of action in the face of uncertainty, and this overvaluation results
in the creation as well as the prevention of impairment. This hypothesis, since
it is based on scattered observations, is presented only to point out several
areas where systematic research is needed.

From the point of view of assessing the effectiveness of medical practice,
this hypothesis is probably too general to be used directly. Needed for such
a task are hypotheses concerning the conditions under which error is likely
to occur, the type of error that is likely, and the consequences of each type
of error. Significant dimensions of the amount and type of error and its consequences would appear to be characteristics of the disease, the physician, the
patient, and the organizational setting in which diagnosis takes place. Thus,
for diseases such as pneumonia, which produce almost certain impairment
unless attended and for which a quick and highly effective cure is available,

the hypothesis is probably largely irrelevant. On the other hand, the hypothesis may be of considerable importance for diseases that have a less certain outcome and for which existing treatments are protracted and of uncertain value. Mental disorders and some types of heart disease are cases in point.

The working philosophy of the physician is probably relevant to the predominant type of errors made. Physicians who generally favor active intervention probably make more Type 2 errors than physicians who view their treatments only as assistance for natural bodily reactions to disease. The physician's perception of the personality of the patient may also be relevant; Type 2 errors are less likely if the physician defines the patient as a "crock," a person overly sensitive to discomfort, rather than as a person who ignores or denies disease.

Finally, the organizational setting is relevant to the extent that it influences the relationship between the doctor and the patient. In some contexts, as in medical practice in organizations such as the military or industrial setting, the physician is not so likely to feel personal responsibility for the patient as he would in other contexts, such as private practice. This may be due in part to the conditions of financial remuneration and, perhaps equally important, the sheer volume of patients dependent on the doctor's time. Cultural or class differences may also affect the amount of social distance between doctor and patient and therefore the amount of responsibility that the doctor feels for the patient. Whatever the sources, the more the physician feels personally responsible for the patient, the more likely he is to make a Type 2 error.

To the extent that future research can indicate the conditions that influence the amount, type, and consequences of error, such research can make direct contributions to medical practice. Three types of research seem necessary in order to establish the true risks of impairment associated with common disease signs. First, controlled field trials of treated and untreated outcomes in a normal population would be needed. Second, perhaps in conjunction with these field trials, experimental studies of the effect of suggestion of illness by physicians and others would be necessary to determine the risks of unnecessary entry into the sick role.

Finally, studies of a mathematical nature seem to be called for. Suppose that physicians were provided with the results of the studies suggested here. How could these findings be introduced into medical practice as a corrective to cultural and professional biases in decision-making procedures? One promising approach is the strategy of evaluating the relative utility of alternative courses of action based upon decision theory or game theory (Chernoff and Moses 1959).

Ledley and Lusted (1959) reviewed a number of mathematical techniques that may be applicable to medical decision-making, one of these techniques being the use of the "expected value" equation, which is derived from game theory. Although their discussion pertains to the relative value of two treatment

procedures, it is also relevant, with only slight changes in wording, to determining the expected values of treatment relative to nontreatment. The expected values of two treatments, they say, may be calculated from a simple
expression involving only two kinds of terms: The probability that the diagnosis is correct and the absolute value of the treatment (at its simplest, the
absolute value is the rate of cure for persons known to have the disease).

The "expected value" of a treatment is:

$$E_t = p_s v_s^s + (1 - p_s)v_h^s$$

that is, the expected value E_t of a treatment is the probability p that the patient has the disease, multiplied by the value (or "cost") v of the treatment for
patients who actually have the disease, plus the probability that the patient
does not have the disease $(1 - p)$, multiplied by the value of the treatment for
patients who do not have the disease, where the superscript refers to the way
the patient is treated (s, sick; h, healthy) and the subscript refers to his actual
condition (s, sick; h, healthy).

Similarly, the expected value of nontreatment is

$$E_n = p_s V_s^h + (1 + P_s)V_h^h$$

that is, the expected value E_n of nontreatment is the probability that the patient has the disease multiplied by the value (or "cost") of treating a person
as healthy who is actually sick, plus the probability that the patient does not
have the disease, multiplied by the value of not treating a healthy person.

The best course of action is indicated by comparing the magnitude of E_t
and E_n. If E_t is larger, treatment is indicated. If E_n is larger, nontreatment is indicated. Evaluating these equations involves estimating the probability of
correct diagnosis and constructing a payoff matrix for the values of v_s^s (proportion of patients who actually had the disease who were cured by the
treatment), v_h^s (the cost of treating a healthy person as sick: inconvenience,
working days lost, surgical risks, unnecessary entry into sick role), v_s^h (cost of
treating a sick person as well: a question involving the proportions of persons
who spontaneously recover and the seriousness of results when the disease
goes unchecked), and finally, $v_h{}^h$ (the value of not treating a healthy person:
medical expenses saved, working days, etc.).

To illustrate the use of the equation, Ledley and Lusted assign *arbitrary* absolute values in a case because, as they say, "The decision of value problems
frequently involves intangibles such as moral and ethical standards which
must, in the last analysis, be left to the physician's judgment" (1959, p. 16).
One may argue, however, that it is better to develop a technique for systematically determining the absolute values of treatment and nontreatment, crude
though the technique may be, than to leave the problem to the perhaps refined, but nevertheless obscure judgment processes of the physician. Particularly in a matter of comparing the value of treatment and nontreatment, the

problem is to avoid biases in the physician's judgment due to the kind of moral orientation discussed previously.

It is possible, moreover, that the difficulty met by Ledley and Lusted is not that the factors to be evaluated are "intangibles," but that they are expressed in seemingly incommensurate units. How does one weigh the risk of death against the monetary cost of treatment? How does one weigh the risk of physical or social disability against the risk of death? Although these are difficult questions to answer, the idea of leaving them to the physician's judgment is probably not conducive to an understanding of the problem.

Following the lead of the economists in their studies of utility, it may be feasible to reduce the various factors to be weighed to a common unit. How could the benefits, costs, and risks of alternative acts in medical practice be expressed in monetary units? One solution may be to use payment rates in disability and life insurance, which offer a comparative evaluation of the "cost" of death and permanent and temporary disability of various degrees. Although this approach does not include everything that physicians weigh in reaching decisions (pain and suffering cannot be weighed in this framework), it does include many of the major factors. It therefore would provide the opportunity of constructing a fairly realistic payoff matrix of absolute values, which would then allow for the determination of the relative value of treatment and nontreatment using the expected value equation.

Gathering data for the payoff matrix may make it possible to explore an otherwise almost inaccessible problem: the sometimes subtle conflicts of interest between the physician and the patient. Although it is fairly clear that medical intervention is unnecessary in particular cases, and that it is probably done for financial gain (Trussel, Ehrlich, and Morehead 1962), the evaluation of the influence of remuneration on diagnosis and treatment is probably in most cases a fairly intricate matter, requiring precise techniques of investigation. If the payoff were calculated in terms of values to the patient *and* values to the physician, such problems could be explored. Less tangible values such as convenience and work satisfactions could be introduced into the matrix. The following statements by psychiatrists were taken from Hollingshead and Redlich's (1958) study of social class and mental disorder: "Seeing him every morning was a chore; I had to put him on my back and carry him for an hour." "He had to get attention in large doses, and this was hard to do." "The patient was not interesting or attractive; I had to repeat, repeat, repeat." "She was a poor unhappy, miserable woman—we were worlds apart" (p. 344).

This study strongly suggests that psychiatric diagnosis and treatment are influenced by the payoff for the psychiatrist as well as for the patient. In any type of medical decision, the use of the expected value equation may show the extent of the conflict of interest between the physician and patient and thereby shed light on the complex process of medical decision-making.

NOTES

1.   An earlier version of this chapter was presented as a paper at the Conference on Mathematical Models in the Behavioral Sciences, sponsored by the Western Management Science Institute, University of California at Los Angeles, Cambria, California, 1961.

2.   Even though this assumption is widely held, it is vigorously criticized within the medical profession. See, for example, Darley (1959). For a witty criticism of both assumptions, see Ratner (1962).

3.   Cf. Stokes and Dawber (1959)

4.   The Framingham Study is an exception to this statement. Even in this study, however, experimental procedures (random assignment to treatment and nontreatment groups) were not used (Dawber, Moore, and Mann 1957).

5.   Some of the findings of the Purdue Farm Cardiac Project support the position taken in the chapter. It was found, for example, that "iatrogenics" took more health precautions than "hidden cardiacs," suggesting that entry into the sick role can cause more social incapacity than the actual disease does. See Eichorn and Anderson (1962).

7

Negotiating Reality

Notes on Power in the Assessment of Responsibility[1]

This chapter shows the application of labeling ideas to two particular contexts: sessions with clients by a defense lawyer and by a practicing psychiatrist. Labeling concepts are very abstract. In order to understand their implications, it is necessary to observe their effects in concrete, particular events. The labeling that the psychiatrist is doing in the interview below is very subtle; it is not completely articulated in words and is probably outside the awareness of both the patient and the psychiatrist. Yet its effects are very constraining. The normalization being practiced by the defense lawyer is also mostly nonverbal. In his case, however, he is probably aware of what he is doing. This chapter provides a very detailed and explicit contrast between the processes of labeling and normalization.

The use of interrogation to reconstruct parts of an individual's past history is a common occurrence in human affairs. Reporters, jealous lovers, and policemen on the beat are often faced with the task of determining events in another person's life and the extent to which he was responsible for those events. The most dramatic use of interrogation to determine responsibility is in criminal trials. As in everyday life, criminal trials are concerned with both act and intent. Courts, in most cases, first determine whether the defendant performed a legally forbidden act. If it is found that he did so, the court then must decide whether he was "responsible" for the act. Reconstructive work of this type goes on less dramatically in a wide variety of other settings, as well. The social worker determining a client's eligibility for unemployment compensation, for example, seeks not only to establish that the client actually is unemployed, but that he has actively sought employment (i.e., that he himself is not responsible for being out of work).

This chapter contrasts two perspectives on the process of reconstructing past events for the purpose of fixing responsibility. The first perspective stems from the commonsense notion that interrogation, when it is sufficiently skillful, is essentially neutral. Responsibility for past actions can be fixed absolutely and independently of the method of reconstruction. This perspective is held by the typical member of society, engaged in his day-to-day tasks. It is also held, in varying degrees, by most professional interrogators. The basic working doctrine is one of *absolute* responsibility. This point of view actually entails the comparison of two different kinds of items: first, the fixing of actions and intentions, and second, comparing these actions and intentions to some predetermined criteria of responsibility. The basic premise of the doctrine of absolute responsibility is that both actions and intentions, on the one hand, and the criteria of responsibility, on the other, are absolute in that they can be assessed independently of social context.[2]

An alternative approach follows from the sociology of knowledge. From this point of view, the reality within which members of society conduct their lives is largely of their own construction.[3] Since much of reality is a construction, there may be multiple realities, existing side by side, in harmony or in competition. It follows, if one maintains this stance, that the assessment of responsibility involves the construction of reality by members: construction both of actions and intentions, on the one hand, and of criteria of responsibility, on the other. The former process, the continuous reconstruction of the normative order, has long been the focus of sociological concern.[4] The discussion in this chapter is limited, for the most part, to the former process, the way in which actions and intentions are constructed in the act of assessing responsibility.

My purpose is to argue that responsibility is at least partly a product of social structure. The alternative to the doctrine of absolute responsibility is that of relative responsibility: The assessment of responsibility always includes a process of negotiation. In this process, responsibility is in part constructed by the negotiating parties. To illustrate this thesis, excerpts from two dialogues of negotiation will be discussed: a real psychotherapeutic interview and an interview between a defense attorney and his client, taken from a work of fiction. Before presenting these excerpts, it is useful to review some prior discussions of negotiation, the first in courts of law, the second in medical diagnosis.[5]

The negotiation of pleas in criminal courts, sometimes referred to as "bargain justice," has been frequently noted by observers of legal processes.[6] The defense attorney or (in many cases, apparently) the defendant himself strikes a bargain with the prosecutor—a plea of guilty will be made provided that the prosecutor will reduce the charge. For example, a defendant arrested on suspicion of armed robbery may arrange to plead guilty to the charge of unarmed robbery. The prosecutor obtains ease of conviction from the bargain, the defendant, leniency.

Although no explicit estimates are given, it appears from observers' reports that the great majority of criminal convictions are negotiated. Newman (1966) states:

> A major characteristic of criminal justice administration, particularly in jurisdictions characterized by legislatively fixed sentences, is charge reduction to elicit pleas of guilty. Not only does the efficient functioning of criminal justice rest upon a high proportion of guilty pleas, but plea bargaining is closely linked with attempts to individualize justice, to obtain certain desirable conviction consequences, and to avoid undesirable ones such as "undeserved" mandatory sentences. (p. 76)

It would appear that the bargaining process is accepted as routine. In the three jurisdictions Newman studied, there were certain meeting places where the defendant, his client, and a representative of the prosecutor's office routinely met to negotiate the plea. It seems clear that in virtually all but the most unusual cases, the interested parties expected to and actually did negotiate the plea.

From these comments on the routine acceptance of plea bargaining in the courts, one may expect that this process would be relatively open and unambiguous. Apparently, however, there is some tension between the fact of bargaining and moral expectations concerning justice. Newman refers to this tension by citing two contradictory statements: an actual judicial opinion, "Justice and liberty are not the subjects of bargaining and barter"; and an off-the-cuff statement by another judge, "All law is compromise." A clear example of this tension is provided by an excerpt from a trial and Newman's comments on it:

> The following questions were asked of a defendant after he had pleaded guilty to unarmed robbery when the original charge was armed robbery. This reduction is common, and the judge was fully aware that the plea was negotiated:
>
> **Judge:**   You want to plead guilty to robbery unarmed?
> **Defendant:** Yes, Sir.
> **Judge:**   Your plea of guilty is free and voluntary?
> **Defendant:** Yes, Sir.
> **Judge:**   No one has promised you anything?

Defendant:	No.
Judge:	No one has induced you to plead guilty?
Defendant:	No.
Judge:	You're pleading guilty because you are guilty?
Defendant:	Yes.
Judge:	I'll accept your plea of guilty to robbery unarmed and refer it to the probation department for a report and for sentencing Dec. 28. (p. 83)

The delicacy of the relationship between appearance and reality is apparently confusing, even for the sociologist-observer. Newman's comment on this exchange has an Alice-in-Wonderland quality: "This is a routine procedure designed to satisfy the statutory requirement and is not intended to disguise the process of charge reduction" (ibid.). If we put the tensions between the different realities aside for the moment, we can say that there is an explicit process of negotiation between the defendant and the prosecution that is a part of the legal determination of guilt or innocence or, in the terms used here, the assessment of responsibility.

In medical diagnosis, a similar process of negotiation occurs but is much less self-conscious than plea bargaining. The English psychoanalyst Michael Balint (1957) refers to this process as one of "offers and responses":

> Some of the people who, for some reason or other, find it difficult to cope with problems of their lives resort to becoming ill. If the doctor has the opportunity of seeing them in the first phases of their being ill, i.e. before they settle down to a definite "organized" illness, he may observe that the patients, so to speak, offer or propose various illnesses, and that they have to go on offering new illnesses until between doctor and patient an agreement can be reached resulting in the acceptance by both of them of one of the illnesses as justified. (p. 18)

Balint gives numerous examples indicating that patients propose reasons for their coming to the doctor that are rejected, one by one, by the physician, who makes counterproposals until an "illness" acceptable to both parties is found. If "definition of the situation" is substituted for "illness," Balint's ob-servations become relevant to a wide variety of transactions, including the kind of interrogation just discussed. The fixing of responsibility is a process in which the client offers definitions of the situation to which the interroga-tor responds. After a series of offers and responses, a definition of the situation acceptable to both the client and the interrogator is reached.

Balint has observed that the negotiation process leads physicians to influ-ence the outcome of medical examinations independently of the patient's condition.[7] He refers to this process as the "apostolic function" of the doc-tor, arguing that the physician induces patients to have the kind of illness that the physician thinks is proper:

Apostolic mission or function means in the first place that every doctor has a vague, but almost unshakably firm, idea of how a patient ought to behave when ill. Although this idea is anything but explicit and concrete, it is immensely powerful, and influences, as we have found, practically every detail of the doctor's work with his patients. It was almost as if every doctor had revealed knowledge of what was right and what was wrong for patients to expect and to endure, and further, as if he had a sacred duty to convert to his faith all the ignorant and unbelieving among his patients. (216)

Implicit in this statement is the notion that interrogator and client have unequal power in determining the resultant definition of the situation. The interrogator's definition of the situation plays an important part in the joint definition of the situation that is finally negotiated. Moreover, his definition is more important than the client's in determining the final outcome of the negotiation, principally because he is well-trained, secure, and self-confident in his role in the transaction, whereas the client is untutored, anxious, and uncertain about his role. Stated simply, the subject, because of these conditions, is likely to be susceptible to the influence of the interrogator.

Note that plea bargaining and the process of "offers and responses" in diagnosis differ in the degree of self-consciousness of the participants. In plea bargaining, the process is at least partly visible to the participants themselves. There appears to be some ambiguity about the extent to which the negotiation is morally acceptable to some of the commentators, but the parties to the negotiations appear to be aware that bargaining is going on and accept the process as such. The bargaining process in diagnosis, however, is much more subterranean. Certainly, neither physicians nor patients recognize the offers and responses process as being bargaining. There is no commonly accepted vocabulary for describing diagnostic bargaining, such as there is in the legal analogy (e.g., "copping out" or "copping a plea"). It may be that in legal processes there is some appreciation of the different kinds of reality [i.e., the difference between the public (official, legal) reality and private reality], whereas in medicine, this difference is not recognized.

The discussion so far has suggested that much of reality is arrived at by negotiation. This thesis was illustrated by materials presented on legal processes by Newman and medical processes by Balint. These processes are similar in that they appear to represent clear instances of the negotiation of reality. The instances are different in that the legal bargaining processes appear to be more open and accepted than the diagnostic process. In order to outline some of the dimensions of the negotiation process and to establish some of the limitations of the analyses by Newman and Balint, two excerpts of cases of bargaining will be discussed: the first is taken from an actual psychiatric "intake" interview, the second from a fictional account of a defense lawyer's first interview with his client.

THE PROCESS OF NEGOTIATION

The psychiatric interview discussed is from the first interview in Gill, New-man, and Redlich (1954). The patient is a 34-year-old nurse who feels, as she says, "irritable, tense, depressed." She appears to be saying from the very beginning of the interview that the external situation in which she lives is the cause of her troubles. She focuses particularly on her husband's behavior. She says he is an alcoholic, is verbally abusive, and won't let her work. She feels that she is cooped up in the house all day with her two small children, but that when he is home at night (on the nights when he is at home), he will have nothing to do with her and the children. She intimates, in several ways, that he does not serve as a sexual companion. She has thought of divorce but has rejected it for various reasons (e.g., she is afraid she couldn't take proper care of the children, finance the babysitters). She feels trapped.[8]

In the concluding paragraph of their description of this interview, Gill et al. give this summary:

> The patient, pushed by we know not what or why at the time (the children—somebody to talk to) comes for help apparently for what she thinks of as help with her external situation (her husband's behavior as she sees it). The therapist does not respond to this but seeks her role and how it is that she plays such a role. Listening to the recording it sounds as if the therapist is at first bored and disinterested and the patient defensive. He gets down to work and keeps asking, "What is it all about?" Then he becomes more interested and sympathetic and at the same time very active (participating) and demanding. *It sounds as if she keeps saying "This is the trouble." He says, "No! Tell me the trouble." She says, "This is it!" He says, "No, tell me," until the patient finally says, "Well I'll tell you." Then the therapist says, "Good! I'll help you"* (p. 133; italics added)

From this summary, it is apparent that there is a close fit between Balint's idea of the negotiation of diagnosis through offers and responses and what took place in this psychiatric interview. It is difficult, however, to document the details. Most of the psychiatrist's responses, rejecting the patient's offers, do not appear in the written transcript, but they are fairly obvious as one listens to the recording. Two particular features of the psychiatrist's responses especially stand out: (1) the flatness of intonation in his responses to the patient's complaints about her external circumstances, and (2) the rapidity with which he introduces new topics, through questioning, when she is talking about her husband.

Some features of the psychiatrist's coaching are verbal, however:

T.95:   Has anything happened recently that makes it . . . you feel that . . . ah . . . you're sort of coming to the end of your rope? I mean I wondered what led you . . .

P.95: (Interrupting.) It's nothing special. It's just everything in general.

T.96: What led you to come to a . . .

P.96: (interrupting) It's just that I . . .

T.97: . . . a psychiatrist just now? [1]

P.97: Because I felt that the older girl was getting tense as a result of . . . of my being stewed up all the time.

T.98: Mmmhnn.

P.98: Not having much patience with her.

T.99: Mmmhnn. (short pause) Mmm. And how had you imagined that a psychiatrist could help with this? (short pause) [2]

P.99: Mmm . . . maybe I could sort of get straightened out . . . straighten things out in my own mind. I'm confused. Sometimes I can't remember things that I've done, whether I've done 'em or not or whether they happened.

T.100: What is it that you want to straighten out?
(Pause)

P.100: I think I seem mixed up.

T.101: Yeah? You see that, it seems to me, is something that we really should talk about because . . . ah . . . from a certain point of view somebody might say, "Well now, it's all very simple. She's unhappy and disturbed because her husband is behaving this way, and unless something can be done about that how could she expect to feel any other way." But, instead of that, you come to the psychiatrist, and you say that you think there's something about you that needs straightening out. [3] I don't quite get it. Can you explain that to me? (short pause)

P.101: I sometimes wonder if I'm emotionally grown up.

T.102: By which you mean what?

P.102: When you're married you should have one mate. You shouldn't go around and look at other men.

T.103: You've been looking at other men?

P.103: I look at them, but that's all.

T.104: Mmmhnn. What you mean . . . you mean a grown-up person should accept the marital situation whatever it happens to be?

P.104: That was the way I was brought up. Yes. (sighs)

T.105: You think that would be a sign of emotional maturity?

P.105: No.

T.106: No. So?

P.106: Well, if you rebel against the laws of society you have to take the consequences.

T.107: Yes?

P.107: And it's just that I . . . I'm not willing to take the consequences. I . . . I don't think it's worth it.

T.108: Mmhnn. So in the meantime then while you're in this very difficult situation, you find yourself reacting in a way that you don't like and that you think is . . . ah . . . damaging to your children and yourself? Now what can be done about that?

P.108: (sniffs; sighs) I dunno. That's why I came to see you.

T.109: Yes. I was just wondering what you had in mind. Did you think a psychiatrist could . . . ah . . . help you face this kind of a situation calmly and easily and maturely? [4] Is that it?

P.109:   More or less. I need somebody to talk to who isn't emotionally involved with the family. I have a few friends, but I don't like to bore them. I don't think they should know . . . ah . . . all the intimate details of what goes on.

T.110:   Yeah?

P.110:   It becomes food for gossip.

T.111:   Mmmhnn.

T.112:   Yeah.

T.113:   Mmm.

P.111:   Besides they're in . . . they're emotionally involved because they're my friends. They tell me not to stand for it, but they don't understand that if I put my foot down it'll only get stepped on.

P.112:   That he can make it miserable for me in other ways . . .

P.113:   . . . which he does.

T.114:   Mmmhnn. In other words, you find yourself in a situation and don't know how to cope with it really.

P.114:   I don't.

T.115:   You'd like to be able to talk that through and come to understand it better and learn how to cope with it or deal with it in some way. Is that right?

P.115:   I'd like to know how to deal with it more effectively.

T.116:   Yeah. Does that mean you feel convinced that the way you're dealing with it now . . .

P.116:   There's something wrong of course.

T.116:   . . . something wrong with that. Mmmhnn.

P.117:   There's something wrong with it. (pp. 176–182)

Note that the therapist reminds her *four times*[9] in this short sequence that she has come to see *a psychiatrist*. Since the context of these reminders is one in which the patient is attributing her difficulties to an external situation, particularly her husband, it seems plausible to hear these reminders as subtle requests for analysis of her own contributions to her difficulties. This interpretation is supported by the therapist's subsequent remarks. When the patient once again describes external problems, the therapist tries the following tack:

T.125:   I notice that you've used a number of psychiatric terms here and there. Were you specially interested in that in your training, or what?

P.125:   Well, my great love is psychology.

T.126:   Psychology?

P.126:   Mmmhnn.

T.127:   How much have you studied?

P.127:   Oh (sighs) what you have in your nurse's training, and I've had general psych, child and adolescent psych, and the abnormal psych.

T.128:   Mmmhnn. Well, tell me . . . ah . . . what would you say if you had to explain yourself what is the problem?

P.128: You don't diagnose yourself very well, at least I don't.

T.129: Well you can make a stab at it. (pause) (pp. 186–187)

This therapeutic thrust is rewarded: the patient gives a long account of her early life that indicates a belief that she was not "adjusted" in the past. The interview continues:

T.135: And what conclusions do you draw from all this about why you're not adjusting now the way you think you should?

P.135: Well, I wasn't adjusted then. I feel that I've come a long way, but I don't think I'm still . . . I still don't feel that I'm adjusted.

T.136: And you don't regard your husband as being the difficulty? You think it lies within yourself?

P.136: Oh he's a difficulty all right, but I figure that even . . . ah . . . had . . . if it had been other things that . . . that this probably—this state—would've come on me.

T.137: Oh you do think so?

P.137: (sighs.) I don't think he's the sole factor. No.

T.138: And what are the factors within . . .

P.138: I mean . . .

T.139: . . . yourself?

P.139: Oh it's probably remorse for the past, things I did.

T.140: Like what? (pause) It's lumping' hard to tell, hunh? (short pause) (pp. 192–194)

After some parrying, the patient tells the therapist what he wants to hear. She feels guilty because she was pregnant by another man when her present husband proposed. She cries. The therapist tells the patient she needs and will get psychiatric help, and the interview ends, the patient still crying. The negotiational aspects of the process are clear: After the patient has spent most of the interview blaming her current difficulties on external circumstances, she tells the therapist a deep secret about which she feels intensely guilty. The patient, and not the husband, is at fault. The therapist's tone and manner change abruptly. From being bored, distant, and rejecting, he becomes warm and solicitous. Through a process of offers and responses, the therapist and patient have, by implication, negotiated a shared definition of the situation— the patient, not the husband, is responsible.

A CONTRASTING CASE

The negotiation process can, of course, proceed on the opposite premise, namely that the client is not responsible. An ideal example would be an interrogation of a client by a skilled defense lawyer. Unfortunately, I have been unable to locate a verbatim transcript of a defense lawyer's initial interview with his client. There is available, however, a fictional portrayal of such an interview, written by a man with extensive experience as defense lawyer, prosecutor, and judge. The excerpt to follow is taken from the novel, *Anatomy of a Murder* (Traver 1958).

The defense lawyer, in his initial contact with his client, briefly questions him regarding his actions on the night of the killing. The client states that he discovered that the deceased, Barney Quill, had raped his wife; he then goes on to state that he then left his wife, found Quill, and shot him:

> "How long did you remain with your wife before you went to the hotel bar?" "I don't remember." "I think it is important, and I suggest you try." After a pause. "Maybe an hour." "Maybe more?" "Maybe." "Maybe less?" "Maybe."
>
> I paused and lit a cigar. I took my time. I had reached a point where a few wrong answers to a few right questions would leave me with a client—if I took his case—whose cause was legally defenseless. Either I stopped now and begged off and let some other lawyer worry over it or I asked him the few fatal questions and let him hang himself. Or else, like any smart lawyer, I went into the Lecture. I studied my man, who sat as inscrutable as an Arab, delicately fingering his Ming holder, daintily sipping his dark mustache. He apparently did not realize how close I had him to admitting that he was guilty of first degree murder, that is, that he "feloniously, willfully and of his malice aforethought did kill and murder one Barney Quill." The man was a sitting duck. (p. 43)

The lawyer here realizes that his line of questioning has come close to fixing the responsibility for the killing on his client. He therefore shifts his ground by beginning "the Lecture":

> The Lecture is an ancient device that lawyers use to coach their clients so that the client won't quite know he has been coached and his lawyer can still preserve the face-saving illusion that he hasn't done any coaching. For coaching clients, like robbing them, is not only frowned upon, it is downright unethical and bad, very bad. Hence the Lecture, an artful device as old as the law itself, and one used constantly by some of the nicest and most ethical lawyers in the land. "Who, me? I didn't tell him what to say," the lawyer can later comfort himself. "I merely explained the law, see." It is a good practice to scowl and shrug here and add virtuously: "That's my duty, isn't it?"
>
> . . . "We will now explore the absorbing subject of legal justification or excuse," I said.
>
> . . . "Well, take self-defense," I began. "That's the classic example of justifiable homicide. On the basis of what I've so far heard and read about your case I do not think we need pause too long over that. Do you?"
>
> "Perhaps not," Lieutenant Manion conceded. "We'll pass it for now."
>
> "Let's," I said dryly. "Then there's the defense of habitation, defense of property, and the defense of relatives or friends. Now there are more ramifications

to these defenses than a dog has fleas, but we won't explore them now. I've already told you at length why I don't think you can invoke the possible defense of your wife. When you shot Quill her need for defense had passed. It's as simple as that."

"Go on," Lieutenant Manion said, frowning.

"Then there's the defense of a homicide committed to prevent a felony—say you're being robbed—; to prevent the escape of the felon—suppose he's getting away with your wallet—; or to arrest a felon—you've caught up with him and he's either trying to get away or has actually escaped." . . .

. . . "Go on, then; what are some of the other legal justifications or excuses?"

"Then there's the tricky and dubious defense of intoxication. Personally I've never seen it succeed. But since you were not drunk when you shot Quill we shall mercifully not dwell on that. Or were you?"

"I was cold sober. Please go on."

"Then finally there's the defense of insanity." I paused and spoke abruptly, airily: "Well, that just about winds it up." I arose as though making ready to leave.

"Tell me more."

"There is no more." I slowly paced up and down the room.

"I mean about this insanity."

"Oh, insanity," I said, elaborately surprised. It was like luring a trained seal with a herring. "Well, insanity, where proven, is a complete defense to murder. It does not legally justify the killing, like self-defense, say, but rather excuses it." The lecturer was hitting his stride. He was also on the home stretch. "Our law requires that a punishable killing—in fact, any crime—must be committed by a sapient human being, one capable, as the law insists, of distinguishing between right and wrong. If a man is insane, legally insane, the act of homicide may still be murder but the law excuses the perpetrator."

Lieutenant Manion was sitting erect now, very still and erect. "I see—and this—this perpetrator, what happens to him if he should—should be excused?"

"Under Michigan law—like that of many other states—if he is acquitted of murder on the grounds of insanity it is provided that he must be sent to a hospital for the criminally insane until he is pronounced sane." . . .

Then he looked at me. "Maybe," he said, "maybe I was insane." . . .

Thoughtfully: "Hm . . . Why do you say that?"

"Well, I can't really say," he went on slowly. "I—I guess I blacked out. I can't remember a thing after I saw him standing behind the bar that night until I got back to my trailer."

"You mean—you mean you don't remember shooting him?" I shook my head in wonderment.

"Yes, that's what I mean."

"You don't even remember driving home?"

"No."

"You don't remember threatening Barney's bartender when he followed you outside after the shooting—as the newspaper says you did?" I paused and held my breath. "You don't remember telling him, 'Do you want some, too, Buster?'?"

The smoldering dark eyes flickered ever so little. "No, not a thing."

"My, my," I said blinking my eyes, contemplating the wonder of it all. "Maybe you've got something there."

The Lecture was over; I had told my man the law; and now he had told me things that might possibly invoke the defense of insanity. (pp. 46–47, 57, 58–59, 60)

The negotiation is complete. The ostensibly shared definition of the situation established by the negotiation process is that the defendant was probably not responsible for his actions.

Let us now compare the two interviews. The major similarity between them is their negotiated character: They both take the form of a series of offers and responses that continue until an offer (a definition of the situation) is reached that is acceptable to both parties. The major difference between the transactions is that one, the psychotherapeutic interview, arrives at an assessment that the client is responsible; the other, the defense attorney's interview, reaches an assessment that the client was not at fault (i.e., not responsible). How can we account for this difference in outcome?

DISCUSSION

Obviously, given any two real cases of negotiation that have different outcomes, one may construct a reasonable argument that the difference is due to the differences between the cases—the finding of responsibility, in one case, and lack of responsibility, in the other, the only outcomes that are reasonably consonant with the facts of the respective cases. Without rejecting this argument, for the sake of discussion only, and without claiming any kind of proof or demonstration, I wish to present an alternative argument; that the difference in outcome is largely due to the differences in technique used by the interrogators. This argument will allow us to suggest some crucial dimensions of negotiation processes.

The first dimension, consciousness of the bargaining aspects of the transaction, has already been mentioned. In the psychotherapeutic interview, the negotiational nature of the transaction seems not to be articulated by either party. In the legal interview, however, certainly the lawyer, and perhaps to some extent the client as well, is aware of and accepts the situation as one of striking a bargain, rather than as a relentless pursuit of the absolute facts of the matter.

The dimension of shared awareness that the definition of the situation is negotiable seems particularly crucial for assessments of responsibility. In both interviews, there is an agenda hidden from the client. In the psychotherapeutic interview, it is probably the psychiatric criterion for acceptance into treatment, the criterion of "insight." The psychotherapist has probably been trained to view patients with "insight into their illness" as favorable candidates for psychotherapy (i.e., patients who accept, or can be led to accept, the problems as internal, as part of their personality, rather than seeing them as caused by external conditions).

In the legal interview, the agenda that is unknown to the client is the legal structure of defenses or justifications for killing. In both the legal and psychiatric cases, the hidden agenda is not a simple one. Both involve fitting abstract and ambiguous criteria (insight, on the one hand, legal justification, on the other) to a richly specific, concrete case. In the legal interview, the lawyer almost immediately broaches this hidden agenda; he states clearly and concisely the major legal justifications for killing. In the psychiatric interview, the hidden agenda is never revealed. The patient's offers during most of the interview are rejected or ignored. In the last part of the interview, her last offer is accepted and she is told that she will be given treatment. In no case are the reasons for these actions articulated by either party.

The degree of shared awareness is related to a second dimension, which concerns the format of the conversation. The legal interview began as an interrogation but was quickly shifted away from that format when the defense lawyer realized the direction in which the questioning was leading the client (i.e., toward a legally unambiguous admission of guilt). On the very brink of such an admission, the defense lawyer stopped asking questions and started, instead, to make statements. He listed the principal legal justifications for killing and, in response to the *client's* questions, gave an explanation of each of the justifications. This shift in format put the client, rather than the lawyer, in control of the crucial aspects of the negotiation. It is the client, not the lawyer, who is allowed to pose the questions, assess the answers for their relevance to his case and, most crucially, to determine for himself the most advantageous tack to take. Control of the definition of the situation—the evocation of the events and intentions relevant to the assessment of the client's responsibility for the killing—was given to the client by the lawyer. The resulting client-controlled format of negotiation gives the client a double advantage. It not only allows the client the benefit of formulating his account of actions and intentions in their most favorable light, it also allows him to select, out of a diverse and ambiguous set of normative criteria concerning killing, the criterion that is most favorable to his own case.

Contrast the format of negotiation used by the psychotherapist. The form is consistently that of interrogation. The psychotherapist poses the questions; the patient answers. The psychotherapist then has the answers at his disposal. He may approve or disapprove, accept or reject, or merely ignore them. Throughout the entire interview, the psychotherapist is in complete control of the situation. Within this framework, the tactic that the psychotherapist uses is to reject the patient's "offers" that her husband is at fault, first by ignoring them, later, and ever more insistently, by leading her to define the situation as one in which she is at fault. In effect, what the therapist does is to reject her offers and to make his own counteroffers.

These remarks concerning the relationship between technique of interrogation and outcome suggest an approach to assessment of responsibility somewhat different from that usually followed. The commonsense approach to interrogation is to ask how accurate and fair is the outcome. Both Newman's and Balint's analyses of negotiation raise this question. Both presuppose that there is an objective state of affairs that is independent of the technique of assessment. This is quite clear in Newman's discussion, as he continually refers to defendants who are "really" or "actually" guilty or innocent.[10] The situation is less clear in Balint's discussion, although occasionally he implies that certain patients are really physically healthy but psychologically distressed.

The type of analysis suggested by this chapter seeks to avoid such presuppositions. It can be argued that *independently* of the facts of the case, the technique of assessment plays a part in determining the outcome. In particular, one can avoid making assumptions about actual responsibility by utilizing a technique of textual criticism of a transaction. The key dimension in such work would be the relative power and authority of the participants in the situation.[11]

As an introduction to the way in which power differences between interactants shape the outcome of negotiations, let us take as an example an attorney in a trial dealing with "friendly" and "unfriendly" witnesses. A friendly witness is a person whose testimony will support the definition of the situation the attorney seeks to convey to the jury. With such a witness the attorney does not employ power but treats him as an equal. His questions to such a witness are open and allow the witness considerable freedom. The attorney may frame a question such as, "Could you tell us about your actions on the night of . . . ?"

The opposing attorney, however, interested in establishing his own version of the witness's behavior on the same night, would probably approach the task quite differently. He may say: "You felt angry and offended on the night of . . . , didn't you?" The witness frequently will try to evade so direct a question with an answer like: "Actually, I had started to . . . " The attorney quickly interrupts, addressing the judge: "Will the court order the witness to respond to the question, yes or no?" That is to say, the question posed by the opposing attorney is abrupt and direct. When the witness attempts to answer indirectly, and at length, the attorney quickly invokes the power of the court to coerce the witness to answer as he wishes, directly. The witness and the attorney are not equals in power; the attorney uses the coercive power of the court to force the witness to answer in the manner desired.

The attorney confronted by an "unfriendly" witness wishes to control the format of the interaction, so that he can retain control of the definition of the situation that is conveyed to the jury. It is much easier for him to neutralize an opposing definition of the situation if he retains control of the interrogation format in this manner. By allowing the unfriendly witness to respond only by "yes" or "no" to his own verbally conveyed account, he can suppress the ambient details of the opposing view that may sway the jury, and thus maintain an advantage for his definition over that of the witness.

In the psychiatric interview just discussed, the psychiatrist obviously does not invoke a third party to enforce his control of the interview. But to impress the patient that she is not to be his equal in the interview he does use a device that is reminiscent of the attorney with an unfriendly witness. The device is to pose abrupt and direct questions to the patient's open-ended accounts, implying that the patient should answer briefly and directly; and, through that implication, the psychiatrist controls the whole transaction. Throughout most of the interview, the patient seeks to give detailed accounts of her behavior and her husband's, but the psychiatrist almost invariably counters with a direct and, to the patient, seemingly unrelated question.

The first instance of this procedure occurs at T.6, the psychiatrist asking the patient, "What do you do?" She replies "I'm a nurse, but my husband won't let me work." Rather than responding to the last part of her answer, which would be expected in conversation between equals, the psychiatrist asks another question, changing the subject: "How old are you?" This pattern continues throughout most of the interview. The psychiatrist appears to be trying to teach the patient to follow his lead. After some 30 or 40 exchanges of this kind, the patient apparently learns her lesson; she cedes control of the transaction completely to the therapist, answering briefly and directly to direct questions and elaborating only on cue from the therapist. The therapist thus implements his control of the interview not by direct coercion but by subtle manipulation.

All of the foregoing discussion concerning shared awareness and the format of the negotiation suggests several propositions regarding control over the definition of the situation. The professional interrogator, whether lawyer or psychotherapist, can maintain control if the client cedes control to him because of his authority as an expert, because of his manipulative skill in the transaction, or merely because the interrogator controls access to something the client wants (e.g., treatment or a legal excuse). The propositions are:

Proposition 1a: *Shared awareness of the participants that the situation is one of negotiation. (The greater the shared awareness the more control the client gets over the resultant definition of the situation.)*

Proposition 1b: *Explicitness of the agenda. (The more explicit the agenda of the transaction, the more control the client gets over the resulting definition of the situation.)*

Proposition 2a: *Organization of the format of the transaction, offers and responses. (The party to a negotiation who responds, rather than the party who makes the offers, has relatively more power in controlling the resultant shared definition of the situation.)*

Proposition 2b: *Counteroffers. (The responding party who makes counteroffers has relatively more power than the responding party who limits his response to merely accepting or rejecting the offers of the other party.)*

Proposition 2c: *Directness of questions and answers. (The more direct the questions of the interrogator and the more direct the answers he demands and receives, the more control he has over the resultant definition of the situation.)*

These concepts and hypotheses are only suggestive until such times as operational definitions can be developed. Although such terms as offers and responses seem to have an immediate applicability to most conversation, it is likely that a thorough and systematic analysis of any given conversation would show the need for clearly stated criteria of class inclusion and exclusion. Perhaps a good place for such research would be in the transactions for assessing responsibility previously discussed. Since some 90% of all criminal convictions in the United States are based on guilty pleas, the extent to which techniques of interrogation subtly influence outcomes would have immediate policy implication. There is considerable evidence that interrogation techniques influence the outcome of psychotherapeutic interviews also. Research in both of these areas would probably have implications for both the theory and practice of assessing responsibility.

CONCLUSION: NEGOTIATION IN SOCIAL SCIENCE RESEARCH

More broadly, the application of the sociology of knowledge to the negotiation of reality has ramifications that may apply to all of social science. The interviewer in a survey or the experimenter in a social-psychological experiment is also involved in a transaction with a client—the respondent or subject. Studies by Rosenthal (1966) and Friedman (1967) strongly suggest that the findings in such studies are negotiated, and influenced by the format of the study.[12] Rosenthal's review of bias in research suggests that such bias is produced by a pervasive and subtle process of interaction between the investigator and his source of data. Those errors that arise because of the investigator's influence over the subject (the kind of influence discussed in this chapter as arising out of power disparities in the process of negotiation) Rosenthal calls "expectancy effects." In order for these errors to occur, there must be direct contact between the investigator and the subject.

A second kind of bias Rosenthal refers to as "observer effects." These are errors of perception or reporting which do not require that the subject be influenced by investigation. Rosenthal's review leads one to surmise that even with techniques that are completely unobtrusive, observer error could be quite large.[13]

The occurrence of these two kinds of bias poses an interesting dilemma for the lawyer, psychiatrist, and social scientist. The investigator of human phenomena is usually interested in more than a sequence of events; he wants to know why the events occurred. Usually this quest for an explanation leads him to deal with the motivation of the persons involved. The lawyer, clinician, social psychologist, or survey researcher tries to elicit motives directly by questioning the participants. But in the process of questioning, as previously suggested, he himself becomes involved in the process of negotiation, perhaps subtly influencing the informants through expectancy effects. A historian, on the other hand, may try to use documents and records to determine motives. He would certainly avoid expectancy effects in this way, but since he would not elicit motives directly, he might find it necessary to collect and interpret various kinds of evidence that are only indirectly related, at best, to determine motives of the participants. Thus, through his choice in the selection and interpretation of the indirect evidence, he may be as susceptible to error as the interrogator, survey researcher, or experimentalist—his error being due to observer effects, however, rather than expectancy effects.

The application of the ideas outlined here to social and psychological research needs to be developed. The five propositions suggested may be used, for example, to estimate the validity of surveys using varying degrees of open-endedness in their interview format. If some technique could be developed that would yield an independent assessment of validity, it might be possible to demonstrate, as Aaron Cicourel has suggested, the more reliable the technique, the less valid the results.

The influence of the assessment itself on the phenomena to be assessed appears to be a ubiquitous process in human affairs, whether in ordinary daily life, in the determination of responsibility in legal or clinical interrogation, or in most types of social science research. The sociology of knowledge perspective, which suggests that people go through their lives constructing reality, offers a framework within which the negotiation of reality can be seriously and constructively studied. This chapter suggests some of the avenues of the problem that may require further study. The prevalence of the problem in most areas of human concern recommends it to our attention as a substantial field of study, rather than as an issue that can be ignored or, alternatively, be taken as the proof that rigorous knowledge of social affairs is impossible.

NOTES

1.   The author wishes to acknowledge the help of the following persons who criticized earlier drafts: Aaron Cicourel, Donald Cressey, Joan Emerson, Erving Goffman,

Michael Katz, Lewis Kurke, Robert Levy, Sohan Lal Sharma, and Paul Webben. The chapter was written during a fellowship provided by the Social Science Institute, University of Hawaii.

2.   The doctrine of absolute responsibility is clearly illustrated in psychiatric and legal discussions of the issue of "criminal responsibility" (i.e., the use of mental illness as an excuse from criminal conviction). An example of the assumption of absolute criteria of responsibility is found in the following quotation: "The finding that someone is criminally responsible means to the psychiatrist that the criminal must change his behavior before he can resume his position in society. *This injunction is not dictated by morality, but so to speak, by reality*" (Sachar 1963; emphasis added).

3.   Cf. Berger and Luckmann (1966).

4.   The classic treatment of this issue is found in Durkheim (1915).

5.   A sociological application of the concept of *negotiation*, in a different context, is found in Strauss et al. (1963, pp. 147–169).

6.   Newman (1966) reports a study in this area, together with a review of earlier work, in "The Negotiated Pleas," Part 3 of the complete work.

7.   A description of the negotiations between patients in a tuberculosis sanitarium and their physicians is found in Roth (1963, pp. 48–59). Obviously, some cases are more susceptible to negotiation than others. Balint implies that the great majority of cases in medical practice are negotiated.

8.   Since this interview is complex and subtle, the reader is invited to listen to it himself and compare his conclusions with those discussed here. The recorded interview is available on the first LP that accompanies Gill, Newman, and Redlich (1954).

9.   Numbers in brackets added.

10.   In his foreword, the editor of the series, Frank J. Remington, comments on one of the slips that occurs frequently, the "acquittal of the guilty," noting that this phrase is contradictory from the legal point of view. He goes on to say that Newman is well aware of this but uses the phrase as a convenience. Needless to say, both Remington's comments and mine can be correct: The phrase is used as a convenience, but it also reveals the author's presuppositions.

11.   Berger and Luckmann also emphasize the role of power, but at the societal level: "The success of particular conceptual machineries is related to the power possessed by those who operate them. The confrontation of alternative symbolic universes implies a problem of power—which of the conflicting definitions of reality will be 'made to stick' in the society" (p. 100). Haley's (1959) discussions of control in psychotherapy are also relevant. See also Haley (1969), "The Power Tactics of Jesus Christ."

12.   Friedman, reporting a series of studies of expectancy effects, seeks to put the results within a broad sociological framework.

13.   Critics of "reactive techniques" often disregard the problem of observer effects. See, for example, Webb, Campbell, Schwartz, and Sechrest (1966).

IV

THE EMOTIONAL/RELATIONAL WORLD

8

A Psychiatric Interview

Alienation between Patient and Psychiatrist[1]

This chapter proposes to enter the emotional/relational world by microanalyzing the details of dialogue. I describe a model of attunement, the state of the social bond, the process through which interactants in the interview fail to achieve joint attention and feeling. Two separate but interrelated systems are involved, a system of communication that can lead to joint attention, and a system of deference that can lead to the sharing of feeling. Through prospective-retrospective and counterfactual methods, interactants appear to use the resources of an entire society in each moment of the encounter. Their ability to understand any given moment in reference to the *extended context* in which it occurs provides the link between the individual and social structure. Society is based on the minute and unexplicated events that make up the *microworld* underlying ordinary discourse. Note that the same psychiatric interview is used in this chapter as in Chapter 7. But here, by analyzing nonverbal cues in addition to the verbal cues used in the earlier chapter, the analysis goes deeper into the web of meaning and emotion spun between the two actors. My analysis uncovers a profound alienation between the psychiatrist and the client, and the shame/rage spiral of helpless anger that both reflects and generates their alienation.

SOCIAL ACTION AND NATURAL LANGUAGE

How are the actions of individuals translated into recurring patterns of collective behavior? How is social structure realized in the actions of individuals? These questions pose an obvious conceptual problem for the social sciences, since they involve the basic model of social behavior. Less obviously, also implicated is the methodology of social science. All empirical research implies a model of social action, since it is ultimately dependent on observations of individual behavior. In the absence of an explicit theory, each researcher is forced to improvise a theory for the case at hand.

I claim that the basic human *bond* involves mental and emotional connectedness, that social organization requires what Stern (1985) has called *attunement* between individuals, the sharing of thoughts and feelings. Society is possible to the extent that its members are able to connect with each other in this way. Society is endangered by anarchy to the extent that interacting members fail to find attunement, lack connectedness, as in the excerpt below. I illustrate this model with findings from recent research, and with a concrete episode of social interaction.

My starting point is an empirical finding from work on artificial intelligence. In the last twenty years an important discovery has been made by attempts at automated interlanguage translation. No algorithm has been found that is sophisticated enough to translate sentences from one natural language to another. To put it in a slightly different way, computers have been unable to understand natural language sentences, and are unlikely to do so in the foreseeable future (Winograd 1984).

As indicated earlier, words in natural languages common words have more than one meaning. Consider the sentence:

The box is in the pen.

Is pen to be understood as an enclosure or as a writing instrument? The computer faced with this decision has recourse only to a dictionary. The native speaker has encyclopedic knowledge of the meaning of pen, and also recourse to contextual knowledge of the sentence involved. Considerations of the usual sizes, shapes, and uses of pens and boxes might lead the native speaker to prefer enclosure as the meaning in this case. Even though this is a relatively simple problem (compared with highly metaphoric sentences) it would be extremely tedious to make the speaker's decision process explicit for just this one sentence.

Even at this elementary level, verbal sentences appear to involve *open*, rather than *closed* domains. The latter involve a finite number of objects, choices, and rules, each of which is uniquely defined. The game of tic-tac-toe provides a simple example: there are only two objects, X and O, and, on the first move, 9 choices. The rules are uniquely defined so that there is no possibility of ambiguity. Most branches of mathematics involve closed domains (e.g., algebra, calculus).

An open domain involves a very large number of objects and rules which are not uniquely defined. The ability to function in an open domain like natural language now appears to be based on extraordinarily complex skills, which are executed with lightning-like rapidity. If we move from the arena of sentences composed of words to those that are spoken, with their accompaniment of nonverbal gestures, we may appreciate the complexity. The amount of information carried by digital language is small compared with that carried by gestures both seen and heard. These gestures are not digital, but continuous; they signal vastly more information.

Findings from conversation and discourse analysis suggest the importance of nonverbal gestures in social interaction (Sacks et al. 1974; Atkinson and Heritage 1984). To summarize many studies, and extrapolate to expected future findings: it would appear that every sentence uttered contains sequencing signals that allow the listener to determine whether the speaker will continue to speak, or stop at the end of the sentence. Although some of this information is conveyed verbally, most is nonverbal. Particularly important is the intonation contour of the sentence: the relative speed, loudness and pitch of the syllables that make it up.

Sequencing signals allow for rapid and seemingly effortless coordination of speech between speakers, a turn-taking system. This finding may constitute the first universal, pan-cultural regularity in language use. Turn-taking also appears to occur virtually at birth in the interaction between caretaker and infant (Stern Hofer, Haft, and Dore 1984; Tronick, Ricks, and Cohn 1982). For this reason it is plausible that the motive and some of the ability to take turns is genetically inherited.

It would appear that sequencing signals are only a minute part of the socially relevant information packed into a spoken sentence. Turn-taking makes up only one small aspect of the *deference/emotion system*. Coordinating turns at speaking is a mechanical problem of avoiding interruption only in part. It also involves a moral issue, the signaling of status.

In order to show respect, the listener must not only avoid speaking before the speaker has finished. There must be a decent pause (perhaps one or two seconds) before the listener begins, showing that speech has been registered, considered. Even if the listener's response has no overlap with the last sentence spoken, the absence of the requisite pause will usually be heard as disrespectful.

The listener must also avoid too lengthy a pause. A silence of more than three or four seconds will usually be heard as implying disagreement or confusion, and therefore as possibly disrespectful. The rhythm of spoken speech is freighted with deference signals. Speaker and listener must both be involved.

In the role of listener, the interactant must take care to detect and honor sequencing signals. In the role of speaker, the signaling task is much greater. Not only must sequencing be signaled, but also the status of the speaker and the listener(s). For example, speaking too rapidly and/or with too little intonation may be understood as signaling lack of interest or respect. Similarly, speaking too slowly and with too much emphasis and gesticulation may also be taken as disrespectful of the listener's ability to understand.

The rhythm of speech is only one of many avenues for awarding or withholding deference. Goffman (1967) proposed that every sentence, its words, paralanguage, and gestures, imply an evaluation of the social and interpersonal status of the interactants:

> The human tendency to use signs and symbols means that evidence of social worth and of mutual evaluations will be conveyed by very minor things, and these things will be witnessed, as will the fact that they have been witnessed. An unguarded glance, a momentary change in tone of voice, an ecological position taken or not taken, can drench a talk with judgmental significance. Therefore, just as there is no occasion of talk in which improper impressions could not intentionally or unintentionally arise, so there is no occasion of talk so trivial as not to require each participant to show serious concern with the way in which he handles himself and the others present. (p. 33)

Goffman argued, furthermore, that all interactants are exquisitely sensitive to the exact amount of deference they are being awarded. If they believe they are receiving too much or, much more frequently, too little, they will be *embarrassed*. His argument concerning embarrassment introduces us into the *realm of feeling*. Before discussing this realm, I once again refer to a second system with which the deference system is entangled.

Goffman's analysis of social interaction also implies another extremely intricate system, the system of communication that enables interactants to understand one another. Although misunderstanding also occurs, it is also clear that interactants, at times, can understand each other. We are certain that we have understood others when we learn that we have correctly predicted their intentions, and they ours.

For example, an appointment is set up on one occasion for dinner on a later one. When our partner arrives at the right time and place, dressed as expected, and in the expected frame of mind, it is clear that interpretive understanding jointly occurred on the earlier occasion. One has correctly understood the other's intent, an inner phenomenon, by noting outer markers. One has understood not only the spoken words, but the inner intent to which the words referred; as expected, the other was not lying or joking. As suggested in the analysis of the excerpt below, the same process of prediction and confirmation can also take place continuously within any given episode.

Although interpretive understanding is so frequent that we take it for granted, it is by no means clear how one "reads another's mind." Goffman (1967) carefully describes the conditions under which successful mind-reading is most likely to occur:

> An understanding will prevail as to when and where it will be permissible to initiate talk, among whom, and by means of what topics of conversation. A set of significant gestures is employed to initiate a spate of communication and as a means for the persons concerned to accredit each other as *legitimate* participants. When this process of *reciprocal ratification* occurs, the persons so ratified are in what might be called "a state of talk"— that is, they have declared themselves officially open to one another for purposes of spoken communication and guarantee together to maintain a flow of words. . . . A *single focus of thought and visual attention,* and a single flow of talk, tends to be maintained and to be legitimated as officially representative of the encounter. (p. 34, emphasis added)

This is a detailed description of the situation in which the "mystic union" of successful communication is likely to occur. The concept of legitimacy that Goffman introduces in this passage serves to bridge the two different systems, deference and communication. Communication occurs most effectively if the interactants "reciprocally ratify" each other as legitimate partners in the communication enterprise. Such ratification is signaled by the virtually continuous awarding and registering of markers of deference. (Bruner 1983, in his analysis of the child's acquisition of language, treats the communication system in a way very similar to Goffman, as the achievement of joint attention, but makes no reference to the deference system.)

It would appear that each uttered sentence is a dynamic package, loaded with an extraordinary amount of information. It may be considered to be analogous to the cell in a living organism, the smallest system. As Goethe suggested in his discussion of morphogenesis, it may be necessary to understand the structure of the cell in order to understand the organism, and the structure of the organism in order to understand the cell. In the proposed model, society exists to the extent that its members are able to achieve attunement, the sharing of meanings and feelings.

EXAMPLE OF INTERACTION RITUAL: THE OPENING EXCHANGE IN A CONVERSATION

Goffman's analysis is so dense and abstract that it is difficult to know whether we understand his meaning. In this section I show, in a concrete example, the markers of deference and communication that suggest the existence of two distinct but interrelated systems. The analysis of this example will be used to describe exchanges of feeling, and the methods interactants (and researchers) use when they are interpreting events.

The passage comes from a widely known psychiatric interview (Gill et al. 1954). It was the basis for a subsequent study (Pittenger, Hockett, and Danehy 1960). Because the original work was accompanied by a long-playing record, Pittenger and his colleagues were able to conduct a microscopic study of the verbal and nonverbal events in the first five minutes of the interview. My analysis of the opening exchange is based upon and further develops that of Pittenger, Hockett, and Danehy (1960). In particular, I use techniques implied in their work, and that of Labov and Fanshel (1977) and Lewis (1971), to interpret the *message stack*. That is, I utilize the words in the transcript and the nonverbal sounds in the recording to infer the unstated implications (the *implicature*) and *feelings* that underlie the dialogue. (For a more detailed discussion, see Scheff 1989.) It begins with the therapist (T) and the patient (P) entering the interviewing room:

T1: Will you sit there. (softly)
P1: (sits down)
T2: (closes doors) What brings you here? (sits down)
P2: (sighs) Everything's wrong I guess. Irritable, tense, depressed. (Sighs) Jus' . . . just everything and everybody gets on my nerves.
T3: Nyeah.
P3: I don't feel like talking right now.
T4: You don't? (short pause) Do you sometimes?
P4: That's the trouble. I get too wound up. If I get started I'm all right.
T5: Nyeah? Well perhaps you will.

A close reading of this passage suggests several puzzles. For example, a pause of *eight seconds* occurs in T4. As already noted, a pause of more than two seconds is likely to make interactants uncomfortable. In seeking to understand why the patient didn't respond to the first part of T4, we notice her preceding comment (P3): "I don't feel like talking right now." Why would the patient not feel like talking when *less than a minute* has elapsed in the interview? I suggest an answer to this question to illustrate Pittenger et al.'s (1960) methods and findings, and my elaboration of them.

Pittenger et al.'s analysis of the language and paralanguage in this passage suggests that failure of attunement occurred during the first three exchanges, resulting in a crisis after T4a. This crisis seems rectified after T4b. Their analysis of the rest of the first five minutes, however, and mine of the rest of the interview, suggest that the crisis was averted only temporarily; the interactants are inadequately attuned for most of the interview. My analysis will be used to illustrate the interdependence of the systems of communication and deference. In this instance, the crisis involved both misunderstanding and an exchange of painful feelings.

Pittenger et al. (1960) suggest that a misunderstanding occurred at T4a because of T's choice of words and intonations in his first three utterances. Almost all of the words chosen are "pronominals," blank checks, and the intonations are "opaque," i.e., flat. P must have heard these utterances, they say, as indicative of detachment, boredom, and disinterest: *"Here we go again! How many times have I heard this kind of thing!"[2] Although unstated, these sentences are implied by the choice of words and intonations, part of the structure of communication that I refer to as implicature.

The authors go on to argue that P has misunderstood at least T's intent, if not his actual behavior. They say that he didn't intend to signal detachment, but neutrality: *"You can tell me anything without fear of condemnation." The authors argue that during the silence after T4a, T must have realized that P had heard him as cold and detached, because in T4b, for the first time, he uses "normal" intonations, i.e., he signals warmth and interest. (Perhaps he also leans forward slightly in his chair, and for the first time, smiles.)

T's understanding of P's mental state is apparently confirmed by P4: she resumes talking. To appreciate the significance of P4, it will be necessary to refer again to the rhythm of turn-taking. P responds to T4 ("You don't?") with an eight-second silence. She does not say *"No, I don't," or its equivalent, signaling that she is still involved. Her silence suggests, rather, that she has withdrawn. Conversation is like a Ping-Pong game. P has put her paddle down on the table, seated herself, and folded her arms. "If you want me to play this game, Buster, you better show me something different than what I have seen so far."

In T4b, T gets the message, and is rewarded with P4. In T5a, however, "Nyeah?" he seems to forget what he just learned, since it is delivered without intonation. This time, however, a silence from P of only 1.8 seconds is necessary to remind him: T5b is delivered with normal intonation.

Another confirmation of the authors' interpretation is suggested by their analysis of the paralanguage of P3 and P4. They say that P seems upset in P3, but not upset in P4. Since the issue of emotional upset will be crucial for my argument, I review and elaborate upon their comments.

EMBARRASSMENT AND ANGER: THE FEELING TRAP OF SHAME-RAGE

Pittenger et al. (1960) interpret the paralanguage of P3 as indicative of *embarrassment* on the patient's part:

> This is a momentary withdrawal of P from the situation into embarrassment with overtones of childishness . . . [as signaled by] the slight oversoft, the breathiness, the sloppiness of articulation, and the incipient embarrassed giggle on the first syllable of *talking*. (1960, p. 30)

Pittenger et al. frequently infer embarrassment in P's utterances, as well as irritation, annoyance, or exasperation. As was the case with the therapist, however, these phenomena do not figure prominently in their concerns, but are only mentioned in passing. The same thing is true of the analysis of emotion that occurs in Labov and Fanshel (1977), even though their analysis is much more sophisticated; for example, they note that signs of the compound emotion "helpless anger" appear very frequently in the patient's paralanguage. Since no explicit theory of the role of emotions in behavior was available to them, these authors made little use of their findings concerning the emotional states of their subjects.

In my analysis, however, their references to emotional states will play a central role. As indicated in earlier chapters, I draw upon the work of Goffman and Lewis to understand the exchanges of feeling that seem to take place in this interview. I will also call upon a graphic depiction of social and psychological process. Kelly et al. (1983) offer a flowchart of processes that take place both within and between interactants, which they call "meshed intrachain sequences." This model can be used to depict a theory of social action. The basic human bond involves both communication and deference, exchanges of thoughts and feelings. It will encompass understanding and misunderstanding, on the one hand, and love and hatred, on the other.

Interpretive understanding (*verstehen*) involves a process between and within interactants that was referred to by G. H. Mead (1934) as "role-taking." He suggested that each party could, under ideal conditions, come very close to sharing the inner experience of the other party. By cycling between *observing* the outer behavior of the other and *imagining* the other's inner experience, a process of successive approximation, intersubjective understanding, can occur. Peirce [1896–1908] used the term "abduction" when describing a similar process in scientists. Scientific discovery, he argued, involves neither induction (observation) nor deduction (imagination) alone, but a very rapid shuttling between the two. This shuttling process can by easily depicted using the Kelly et al. model.

Like Goffman's analysis, the formulations concerning *verstehen* by Dilthey, Mead, Peirce, and others have been so abstract and dense that it is difficult to find out if they are useful or not. Because they offer no applications to concrete episodes, their ideas have remained somewhat mysterious.

Bruner's (1983) work on the acquisition of language is much more concrete. He does not invoke the concept of *verstehen,* but refers rather to "joint attention." His examples of instances in which the mother teaches the baby the meaning of a word suggest the origins of intersubjectivity. The mother places an object (such as a doll) in the baby's line of gaze, shakes it to make sure of the baby's attention, and says "See the pretty *dolly*." The mother intends only to teach the name of the doll, but in doing so, she also teaches the baby shared attention. I will illustrate shared attention with the incident already cited. Before doing so, it is necessary to outline a model of exchanges of feeling.

Goffman's analysis of interaction ritual suggests that embarrassment and anticipation of embarrassment are pervasive in social interaction and, particularly, that they are exchanged *between* the interactants. Lewis's analysis outlines the process of *inner* sequences, how one may be ashamed of being angry, and angry that one is ashamed, for example. The Kelly model allows us to envision the joint occurrence of emotional processes between and within, how love and hate are both psychological and social processes.

Studies of infant-caretaker interaction, particularly that of Stern, Hofer, Haft, and Dore (1984), provide a picture of the elemental love relationship. Beginning very early in the infant's life, perhaps even on the first day, the infant and caretaker begin a process that might be described as falling in love. It seems to begin with taking turns at gazing into the other's eyes. This process rapidly leads to mutual eye gaze, mutual smiling, and what Stern calls mutual delight. Love can be visualized as occurring between and within the mother and child, involving meshed intrachain sequences. The perception of the mother's smile causes the baby to feel delight, which leads it to smile, which causes the mother to feel delight, which leads to a further smile, and so on, a virtuous circle.

The hate relationship can also be delineated, by using Lewis's concept of the feeling trap. A combination of anger and shame snowballs between and within the interactants, leading to an extraordinarily intense and/or long-term relationship of hatred. In the kind of hatred that occurs between avowed enemies, the shame component in the exchange of feelings is not acknowledged, but the anger is overt. The vendetta provides a model for this kind of bond, involving insult to honor (shaming), vengeance in order to remove the stain on honor, and mutual hatred and interminable conflict. As in the love relationship, there is a snowballing of emotional reactions between and within the antagonists: an action of one party that is perceived as hostile by the other leads that other to feel angry and ashamed, which leads to a hostile action, which causes the same cycle in the other party, and so on, a vicious circle. In relationships between intimates, elements of both love and hate often seem to be involved:

> I hate while I love; would you ask how I do it?
> My case proves it true; that's all there is to it.
> (Catullus)

To point out some of the ingredients of this mixture, I return to the exchange that was discussed above.

In this interview there are several instances of attunement between the therapist and the patient. As already indicated, even though they got off to a bad start, between T4b and the end of T5b one such moment occurred. The therapist, in the silence after T4a, seems to have correctly sensed the cause of P's embarrassed withdrawal, and corrected for it. In T4b he offers the sympathy and respect missing from his initial manner. The patient responds appreciatively, relieved of her embarrassment. Such moments recur in the interview, but infrequently. For the most part, the interview is characterized by misunderstandings and feelings like those in the initial crisis at T3–T4a. Since there is little direct hostility or anger expressed, the interview is not an open quarrel, but involves many impasses.

The causes of impasse can be inferred from Pittenger et al.'s (1960) analysis. They do not attempt to characterize the mood of the interview as a whole, but they point to recurring elements in the manner of the two interactants. They repeatedly remark on the therapist's tone: "cold, remote, and detached." They also point repeatedly to the emotionality of the patient. For example, about P6, "I'm a nurse, but my husband won't let me work," they say:

> The narrowed register, overflow, scattered squeeze, and the rasp on "work," together with the [lack of] intonation on the last phrase, mark P6 as a real complaint, invested with *real annoyance, misery, and resentment.* (50–51, emphasis added)

The authors also note frequent instances of embarrassment in the patient's manner (e.g., P70, P101b). Finally, they note several instances of what they call "whining," "fishwifely raucousness" (P82, P83b), or a "fishwifely whine" (P158) (these particular comments seem to slur the patient's gender, social class, and emotionality). In summarizing the therapist's tactics, the authors suggest that one of the therapist's primary goals is to get the patient to reduce her level of emotionality in the session.

The paralanguage that the authors say accompanies the patient's "annoyance," "resentment," "raucousness," and "whining" is very similar to what Labov and Fanshel (1977) take to be the signs of "helpless anger," i.e., shame-anger. At the beginning of the interview, the patient is surprised, puzzled, and very soon insulted by the therapist's manner. Although there are moments of reprieve, the patient seems to remain in that state for most of the interview. Since neither the patient nor the therapist acknowledges her emotional state, the interview turns into a polite but nevertheless baffling impasse, a mixture of understanding and misunderstanding, acceptance and rejection, love and hate.

So far the excerpt from the interview has been used to show the entanglement of communication and deference systems, how in this case misunderstanding and exchanges of embarrassment and anger go hand in hand. The next step is to show how attunement of thought and feeling, or its absence, is related to social structure.

INTERPRETATION AND CONTEXT

Before continuing with the example, it is necessary to outline what I consider to be innovative aspects of Pittenger et al.'s (1960) methodology:

1. the emphasis on paralanguage,
2. the separation of inferences from observations,
3. the prospective-retrospective method of understanding,
4. the use of counterfactual variants.

The decision of the authors to attempt a virtually complete phonemic and phonetic analysis of every word of a text represents a marked departure from not only the practice of everyday life, but also from the practice of research on human behavior. The intensity of their description of the characteristics of the utterances, and of their analysis and interpretation of these characteristics gives their work a microscopic quality. They deal not just with the nuances of communication, but with the nuances of nuances.

The intensity of their analysis in itself results in a somewhat unexpected finding: if one forces oneself to pay as much attention to the paralanguage of a message as to the language, the extraordinary richness and complexity of human actions springs into life off the printed page. The sensation of reading the author's descriptions and interpretations is like looking at a drop of water under a microscope: one is shocked by the seemingly infinite variety of life that suddenly appears below the smooth surface of ordinary experience.

The authors' method of intensive, rather than extensive investigation may hold a lesson for contemporary social science and psychology. Perhaps we have put too much emphasis on generalization, on extensive knowledge, without also understanding a single instance very well. Perhaps the single case, sufficiently understood, could generate hypotheses that would be worth testing. As William Blake had said: "To see a world in a grain of sand."

The second of the authors' methods concerns strict separation between their *observations* of utterances, and the *inferences* they make on the basis of these observations. This principle is made explicit by the authors: they strongly urge research discipline. The researcher must be continually aware, and wary, that interpretations are inferential, only, and therefore have a different status than observations, raw facts in the recorded transaction.

At first glance, this method doesn't seem at all innovative: it merely repeats one of the accepted tenets of science. However, their attempt to honor this tenet turned out to be fruitful, because they were unable to carry it out completely. By considering their analysis to be part of the text that I am investigating (along with the recorded transcript) I make deductions about the *authors'* process of understanding, the process that enabled them to arrive at many of their interpretations.

The authors show varying degrees of tentativeness or confidence in their interpretations. The most tentative are those made at the beginning of their analysis. In their first interpretation of the therapist's utterances, T2 and T3, they use the device of reporting the response of only one of the authors, how these two utterances were heard as cold and detached. This is their most cautious mode. Later, with respect to T16, they provide an interpretation that is less tentative, but still restrained, when they state that by this point, all three of the authors "came to have the feeling" that although there was some variation in T's style, it was basically "cold, detached, and remote."

This latter statement is typical of their usual style of interpretation. The implication is that they are only reporting an inference that could easily be in error. With conventional scientific caution, these statements invite the reader to make his or her own interpretations for the sake of comparison.

There is another style that the authors occasionally use, however, which seems to be a lapse from scientific prudence. These are the occasions in which they state that some matter is obvious, clear, or, in one instance, "unmistakable." These matters are almost always inferences about what one of the interactants understands or intends. Although the authors do not acknowledge it, they are implying, with complete confidence, that they have been able to penetrate into the minds of the persons whose speech they have studied.

In order to illustrate these lapses from their stated rule, here is the evidence they cite for their most unguarded imputation:

> P2b shows unmistakable signs of "rehearsal." In anticipating the interview, P has planned certain things that she is going to say, and now simply reads this one off from memory. (Many therapists put a premium on spontaneity of patient's response during therapy; we must therefore make it clear that in the present context we imply no adverse judgment of P.) The pause with glottal closure after *so,* and then the spacing-out of the three adjectives, the first two with nonfinal intonations and the third with a distinctly final one, are reminiscent of "dramatic reading," and not characteristic of ordinary informal conversation. The wording—particularly the nonuse of *and* between the second and third adjectives—also contributes to the impression.
>
> A sort of pedantic itemization, of which P's rehearsed statement is reminiscent, is customary in schools and in certain other situations where a student or junior is addressing a teacher or other senior. This style is perhaps especially emphasized by doctors. We learn later that P is a nurse. Her experience as a nurse may have reinforced earlier school experience to supply the basis for the pedantic itemizing style; one need only think of a nurse delivering a report on a patient, partly from written notes (*The patient was sleepless, uncomfortable, . . .*). P knows, and has known in advance, that this interview is with a doctor, and knows from experience that the "nurse's report" style is one of the appropriate ways to address a doctor.

Is this evidence strong enough to warrant the authors' disregard for their own methodological principle? After listening to P2b several times, I found their argument compelling. However, the reader is not required to accept my judgment on faith. Since the record of this interview is available in most university libraries (Gill et al. 1954), interested readers can make their own judgment. For this reason, all of the authors' inferences are directly falsifiable, which gives their study a unique evidential status. Perhaps the raw data can serve as a warrant for the *validity* of the findings. The ready availability of the raw data stands in stark contrast to quantitative studies. I return to this issue below, when I consider an appropriate methodology for testing the theory that is offered here.

If we accept the authors' assertion about this utterance, then we are confronting an important issue. The authors are claiming that not only are they are able to share the conscious experience of the person being studied, as they do many times in their analysis, but in this instance, they are able to understand what the patient was thinking before she even arrived on the scene. They attribute to her what Mead called "imaginative rehearsal." Moreover, they are so confident of the validity of their imputation that they seem to forget their own rule, of rigorously separating inference from observation.

Another example of their unguarded style of inference occurs in their analysis of T4: "In either case, *it is clear that P does not understand T,* and the only obvious factor that may possibly be responsible is his intended opaque intonation" (emphasis added in this and the following passage). In the next sentence they also make an impetuous inference with respect to T's experience: "After a silence of eight seconds (which is quite a long time), this [the authors are referring to P not understanding T3] *becomes obvious to T,* and he tries again." In an un-self-conscious way, the authors infer, with great confidence, the inner experience of the interactants at this moment in the session.

Except for these and a few similar lapses, the book is a model of scientific rigor and probity. How can they be explained? To understand the source of these errors, it will be necessary to consider the two further methods that the authors used to interpret the text they studied.

The third of the authors' methods is the prospective-retrospective method of understanding (Schutz 1962). In interpreting the significance of the utterance being considered, the authors do not limit themselves to the immediate context, but range far and wide, backward and forward.

For example, in their analysis of P2, quoted above, the inference that it is rehearsed is based on their knowledge that later in the interview P reveals that she is a nurse. The authors use this piece of information, which is prospective, in a retrospective way: she may have been accustomed, as a nurse, to reporting to doctors in the "pedantic" style they hear in P2. Thus the rehearsal inference is based not merely on the authors' knowledge of events in the text, but also their imagination of P's experiences even before she began this transaction. In interaction, as well as in research on interaction, to understand the significance of an utterance, one must consider not only what is happening at the moment, but also what has happened before, and what might happen in the future.

Although the authors never mention this method, it is a vital element in their analysis. They use it in all of their more extensive interpretations. I have just described one of their many uses to infer a moment of the patient's inner experience. They also use it, again only implicitly, to explain the basis of their own understanding of the text.

For example, they state that by the therapist's sixteenth utterance, all three of them "came to have the feeling" that T's manner to this point in the text was usually "cold, detached, and remote." They explain that it was only at this point in the analysis "that we finally realized that all of us had been registering a certain reaction to T's speech." In retrospect, they had understood they had been having a similar reaction to most of his earlier utterances that they were having to T16. Although not mentioned, their knowledge of T's manner after T16 was probably also involved. The interpretation of T's intonation in T16 utilized, it would seem, the prospective-retrospective method.

They also use this method with their analysis of T16 in a much more wide-ranging way. They state that their "impression of relative coldness is based on a comparison of his interview style with styles of everyday conversation. Perhaps relative to the interview styles of other therapists, T's manner in this interview would be felt as warm" (Pittenger et al. 1960, p. 134). In the first sentence they seem to be saying that they each actually carried out, in their own mind, a comparison of T's style with what each thought of as the style of intonation of the average everyday conversation. In the second sentence they suggest that they did not actually carry out a comparison of T's style with the other therapists that they have known, but if they had, his might have turned out warmer.

Although it is only implicit, I believe that the authors used these two inferences throughout their analysis, in imputing understandings to the two interactants. That is, they used the first inference to imply that the patient must also have heard T's intonations as cold and detached, since her standard of comparison would be not other therapists, but ordinary conversations. (We learn toward the end of the interview that P had seen a psychiatrist only once before the present interview.) They use the second inference to imply that T, on the contrary, might have been hearing his intonation relative to other therapists. This point is hinted at in the authors' analysis of T3 and of T16 ("the special sub-culture of the psychiatric interview").

One might consider these two inferences to be couched in the authors' most completely guarded style of inferential statements, since they are never actually stated (my single jest in these sober pages!). Nevertheless, these inferences overshadow the authors' whole analysis: the two interactants have a misunderstanding about the meaning of T's intonations, since they bring to the transaction two different sets of earlier experiences. The method of prospective-retrospective understanding can be seen to be a powerful tool for reaching interpretive understandings.

The fourth and final of the authors' methods they refer to as the "Working Principle of Reasonable Alternatives." I prefer to call it the method of *counterfactual variants,* in order to relate it to earlier developments in philosophy and social theory. Counterfactuality concerns what might have happened in a given instance, but did not. In human experience, the imagination of what might have happened often seems to be at least as important as what actually happened.

Although Mead (1934) did not use this term, his theory provides a disciplined analysis of the origins of counterfactual imagination in the development of the self, and its importance in social interaction. The movement from the *game stage* to the stage of the *generalized other* is the basis for the human ability to escape from outer stimuli. It lays the foundation for the ability to construct imaginary standpoints, which is necessary for reflective intelligence and the construction of a self. Vaihinger's philosophy of "as if" (1924) explores some of the implications of the ability to live in worlds that are subjunctive, contingent, or conditional.

By far the most comprehensive exploration of this issue can be found in the work of the George Steiner, in his magnum opus, *After Babel* (1975). Although focused on the problems involved in translation from one language to another, Steiner also establishes that *all understanding involves translation, translation from one mind to another.* Every understanding involves "translation" from the personal idiom and cultural background of one person, to the personal idiom and cultural background of another, from one imagined world to another. His discussion of the all but insuperable impediments to communication between men and women, ethnic groups, and social classes exactly parallels his illustrations of the limitless chances for error in interlingual translation.

Counterfactuality is also of fundamental importance in physical and social science, but is virtually undiscussed. Peirce's [1896–1908] concept of abduction implies the critical importance of counterfactuals. Pierce seems to be saying that if the scientist is to come up with an original and important hypothesis, he or she must be just as aware of what is not occurring as what is. One does not observe events passively, but within a framework, a framework that includes counterfactual conditions or expectations.

The prevailing mood in modern science is inductive: one makes discoveries by passively observing nature. According to this view, systematic observation gives rise to generalizations about recurring sequences of events. As suggested, Mead and other theorists of counterfactuality indicated that all human understanding, including scientific understanding, depends upon the imagination, as well as on accurate observations. As suggested, Pittenger and his colleagues not only reacted to the actual utterances they could hear on the tape, but they seem to have understood what was said by placing it in the context of what could have been said but was not. A brief and somewhat begrudging acknowledgment of the importance of counterfactuality in physical science can be found in Hofstadter (1975, pp. 634–640, 641–644).

Pittenger et al. (1960) frequently employed the method of counterfactual variants. In their first analysis of an utterance by T, (T2), they note that three of the four words in "What brings you here?" are "substitutes," words with no actual reference. In order to understand the significance of T2 as uttered, they contrast it with five alternatives that were not uttered: "what *troubles, what *problems, what *difficulties," and, instead of "here," T might have said *"to a psychiatrist" or *"to this clinic." Similarly, in my own comparison of what the authors might have done had they noticed that most of the words in T1 were also substitutes, they might have tried out the sentence "Will you please sit there, Mrs. Johnson, where it will be convenient and comfortable for you?" as a counterfactual alternative to T1. (This is an actual initial sentence used by another therapist, FD2's therapist in Lewis 1971.)

As they did the prospective-retrospective method, the authors use the method of counterfactual variants in every one of their major interpretations at least once. In the case of T2, they use it twice. The first use, quoted above, was to try alternatives involving words that were not substitutes. The second use of the method on T2 was much more elaborate, trying out five variant stress patterns in the sentence, with the greatest stress on "What" for the first variant, on "brings" for the second, and so on. Since T's actual utterance contained a complex pattern of stresses, with ties between two words, and a crucial change in stress from the beginning of the last word to its end, the authors could have tried out many more than five variants.

At first glance it might seem that the method of counterfactual variants, as used by the authors, is laborious beyond any conceivable value it might have. Since I am going to claim that if anything, the authors were too timid, rather than too bold, I will draw some of the implications of their analysis of T2 (and of mine of T1) for an understanding of the emotional exchange between T and P during the first moments of the session.

With respect to T2, the authors make the case that the words used are mostly substitutes, and that they have an opaque intonation. Later in their analysis, they imply that P has misunderstood the meaning that T intended for his intonations, as part of their interpretation of the impact of T's style on P throughout the first five minutes. This is the only use they make of their lengthy analysis of T2. They never refer to the significance of T's use of substitutes at all.

If we wish to understand the emotional components of the exchanges between T and P, we can make further use of the authors' analysis of T2, if we join it with my comments on the similarity between the words used in T1 and T2; most of the words in both sentences were substitutes. Suppose we extend the method of counterfactual variants beyond its uses at the hands of the authors. They limit themselves to imagining words or sentences alternative to those that were used by the therapist (whom I will call Dr. Noland) and the patient, whom I have already called Mrs. Johnson.

Suppose that instead of Mrs. Frank Johnson, the patient had been Mrs. Lyndon Johnson. Is it conceivable that T could have greeted her with these two blank check sentences? ("Will you sit there?" and "What brings you here?") We know that the second sentence was intoned opaquely. Even if we allow that the intonation of T1 might have been more normal than T2, since Gill et al. (1954) tell us that it was spoken softly, the conclusion still seems inescapable, to take on the authors' most impetuous style of inferential statement. Mrs. Lyndon Johnson would have found these two utterances insufferably rude, and would probably have said so, and perhaps would have even bid Dr. Noland a heated farewell. The counterfactual of Mrs. Lyndon Johnson suggests that Mrs. Martha Johnson may also have been insulted by T's manner.

I have drawn upon the authors' analysis of the verbal and nonverbal elements in the early parts of the session to solve the problem of the patient's withdrawal at P3, and the therapist's response to her withdrawal. Their analysis, and my extension of it, suggests that P heard the therapist's first two utterances as cold and detached, to the point of rudeness. She became confused and hurt by this treatment, to the point of withdrawing.

Turning now to their analysis of the therapist's experience of P3, and P's silence after T4a, the authors infer that he must have understood her hearing of his initial utterances as detached, because he changes his manner of intonation in T4b, ("Do you sometimes?") it becomes much more evocative of interest and concern, as in ordinary, as opposed to therapy conversations. Furthermore, they argue, the patient's response in P4 seems to confirm these inferences; she ends her withdrawal, resuming her part in the conversation. Using the authors' analysis and my own, it has been possible to arrive at an understanding of a crisis and its resolution.

It should be noted that the last two of the four methods used by the authors differ in character from the first two. The prospective-retrospective and counterfactual methods are intuitive and freewheeling; they draw upon the resources of the entire culture. In order to understand a particular utterance, Pittenger et al. do not limit themselves to the immediate context, but range far and wide in their imagination, over what could have happened before, during, or after the utterance.

The first two methods, the exhaustive analysis of the text and the separation of observation and inference, are, by contrast, not intuitive but analytical. These methods are used to control and discipline the flight of the imagination. The continuous shuttling back and forth between imaginative and analytic methods, between intuition and observation implied in their narrative, illustrates what Peirce [1896–1908] meant by the method of abduction. If one inter-prets a text that is publicly available, as Peirce did not, the interpretation may be as verifiable as in any other method in science.

IMPLICATURE, CONTEXT, AND SOCIAL STRUCTURE

In this section I suggest a model of the process that links individual behav-ior to social structure, using the Pittenger et al. (1960) study as an example. Since their narrative provides a report not only of their methods and findings but also of their inner experiences, it can be used to envision the complex process of social action. The key concepts in the proposed model are the *message stack,* on the one hand, and the *extended context,* on the other.

The authors understood the intentions of the interactants because they didn't limit themselves to observing their actual utterances, but also imagined their inner experiences. In order to accomplish this feat, the authors referred not only to the interactants' words and nonverbal gestures, but also to their feel-ings and to the "implicature," the unstated implications of their words and gestures.

An example of implicature is the authors' comments on the therapist's choice of pronominals in T3, and the flatness of intonation. *"Here we go again! How many times have I heard this kind of thing before!" This sentence was never actually uttered. It is the meaning that the authors imagine the patient attributed to the words and gestures in T3. The authors constructed this counterfactual implication by shuttling back and forth between the words and gestures they observed before, during, and after this moment, imagining what these words and gestures might have implied to the patient. This is the informal process of testing inferences about inner experience by checking their implications against observable outer signs, the process of role-taking.

Although the authors are extremely energetic in pursuit of the unstated implications of the words and gestures, they are much less so with respect to the fourth component of the message stack, the feelings. Like Labov and Fan-shel (1977), they limit themselves to the inductive method with respect to feelings. They note the occurrence of signs of anger and embarrassment, but do not construct complex inferences with respect to them, as they do with the implicature. Because no theories of emotional process were available to them, both sets of authors emphasize the cognitive components of the inter-action they observed.

Lewis's work on feeling traps, together with the Kelly model, provides a way of integrating all four components of the message stack. The observables, the words and gestures, provide data for making inferences about the inner ex-periences of the interactants, the thoughts and feelings.

The method of inferring implicature plays a crucial role, since it serves as a bridge between observables and inner feelings on the other. If the interactants *stated* the implications of their actual words and gestures, rather than being silent about them, they could probably understand why such intense emotions are aroused by them. Since the interactants do not state them, however, and seldom investigate them, they ignore or are puzzled by the intense *feelings* engendered.

My analysis of the components of the message stack in the interview suggests that the therapist and the patient are seldom attuned because they are enmeshed in a feeling trap. Mutual resentment, puzzlement, and misunderstanding occur because of chain reactions of shame and anger within and between them. The signs of a shame-rage spiral are clear in the patient, her embarrassment and exasperation. They are less obvious in the therapist, however. To clarify this point, it is necessary to return to Lewis's distinction between bypassed and overt, undifferentiated emotion.

My interpretation of the patient's emotional state is that from T3 onwards she is frequently involved in a spiral of *overt*, undifferentiated shame and anger. She is grossly insulted by the therapist's manner. Although she tries to hide her feelings, they can be inferred from her words and gestures, as Pittenger et al. show.

Bypassed emotion does not cause disruption of behavior and speech, as the overt, undifferentiated type does. Rather it disrupts the fine-tuning of thought necessary for effective action in problematic situations. Since one's inner resources are given over to emotional arousal and to the attempt to hide it, one cannot devote full attention to problem-solving. At best, while obsessing because of unacknowledged shame and anger, one can go into a holding pattern, repeating stereotyped behavior sequences.

In the present instance, the therapist does not respond constructively to the impasse between him and the patient. As Pittenger et al. indicate, his agenda appears to be to discourage the patient from her repeated emotional complaints about her husband. Like the patient, he simply repeats the same sequence over and over, even though it is ineffective. He does not attempt to negotiate about their respective agendas: *"I notice that you keep complaining about your husband. Could you get away from him a while, and talk more about yourself?" Similarly, the patient does not say *"I notice that every time I express emotion, you respond by ignoring it and asking me a question about some irrelevant fact. I am puzzled and offended, because you seem to be condemning my feelings just like my husband does. What are you doing?" Since their conflicting agendas are never discussed, they butt heads for the entire interview.

It is possible that the therapist is ineffective because the patient's behavior touches off his own shame-anger sequence. He may have experienced the patient's balking and emotionality as insulting to his authority or, more subtly, to his competence as a therapist. In order to test this hypothesis, it would be necessary to investigate this same therapist's behavior in a different setting, one in which he was acting effectively, to highlight the subtle signs of by-passed shame and rage in the present interview (Scheff 1987).

The inference of enmeshment of the two interactants leads to the last issue to be discussed. In what way are the exchanges of feeling and innuendo that are discussed here related to social structure? The spontaneous use of prospective-retrospective and counterfactual methods by the interactants and by Pittenger et al. (1960), and by Labov and Fanshel (1977), who use very similar methods in their study, suggests an answer to this question.

These methods suggest that in order to understand the meaning of even a single utterance, it may be necessary to invoke not just the immediate *con-text,* but what might be called the *extended context,* i.e., all that has hap-pened before or after, retrospectively and prospectively, and all that might have happened instead, counterfactually. Each interpretation of meaning pre-supposes not only the history of the whole relationship, but also the history of the whole society, insofar as it is known to the interactants. Effective com-munication implies a social structure shared between the interactants. Inso-far as interaction takes place in an open domain such as natural language, and insofar as the interactants are experts in that domain, then each exchange depends upon and helps maintain the social structure.

I have argued that there is a microworld underlying all social interaction. This microworld connects individuals in shared meanings and feelings, and also connects them to the social structure of their society. I have given an ex-ample of analysis of the microworld involved in a single brief exchange be-tween a therapist and his patient. In this example, following Pittenger et al. (1960), I examined the message stack of words, gestures, implicature, and feelings that occurred at several particular moments during the exchange. By interpreting these stacks, we can come to understand the thoughts and feel-ings of the interactants.

According to the theory outlined here, social interaction involves an open domain. In order to understand any given utterance, the interactants must have access to the extended context of the utterance, all events that took place or could have taken place before, during, and after the particular mo-ment. The micromomentary actions of the interactants in relating the moment to the extended context connect them with the social structure. Paradoxically, understanding social structure involves examination of the minute events in the microworld.

The methodology appropriate to testing such a theory requires painstak-ing analysis of recorded instances of social interaction: the repeated playing of film or audiotape allows the researcher to use the same intuitive interpre-tation of the message stack that is used by the interactants. I have argued, in another place, that the reporting of this kind of study would require that the recorded text be appended, so that the readers could also use their own intuitive expertise in assessing the validity of the findings (Scheff 1997). A method like this would bridge the present gap between the proponents of objective measurement and those who uphold intuitive methods, perhaps helping to resolve what are usually thought of as irreconcilable differences.

This chapter and the next suggest that the emotional/relational world, usually invisible, can be made visible, if we play close enough attention to the details of discourse. The discourse in this chapter suggests a profound alienation between a patient and a psychiatrist. The discourse in the next chapter suggests that a skillful psychotherapist can bridge the gap, building a secure bond with a profoundly alienated patient.

NOTES

1. This chapter is largely based on Chapter 6 in my 1990 book. The earliest version was indebted to conversations with Ursula Mahlendorf and Suzanne Retzinger.

2. The asterisk (*) is used in linguistics to signal an imagined statement, one that did not actually occur, a "counterfactual."

9

Labeling in the Family
Hidden Shame and Anger

The analysis of details of the dialogue of therapy sessions suggests that my earlier labeling theory of mental illness can be enriched by including discourse analysis at a microlevel. The session that I use to illustrate this point is between an anorexic woman and her therapist. Discourse analysis shows how unacknowledged shame can be a cause of both primary and secondary deviance. In family systems, it causes primary deviance, and in the interaction between the family and the community, it causes secondary deviance. The dialogue suggests that the family labeling process is subtle and outside awareness. In the anorexic patient's family, stigmatization is a two-way street: through innuendo, all the family members—including the patient—surreptitiously attack each other. But only the patient's violence has an overt component. Like the family members, she attacks others through innuendo, but she also starves herself. All the others use only emotional violence. Since the violence of the family is hidden, it is the patient who was formally labeled.

In this chapter I introduce a new theory and method, which leads to modification of my earlier work on labeling in mental illness. I consider myself lucky to be able to criticize my own original formulation (1966; 1984), because when I criticize the work of others, they often take it personally. In criticizing my own work, I am free to view the criticism in its most favorable light, perhaps as a sign of intellectual growth, rather than showing how inadequate the original formulation was. Like most other theories of human behavior, the original theory was highly specialized, yet insufficiently detailed. It was specialized since it dealt behaviorally with social structure/process. It omitted most inner events, both those concerning mental illness and those concerning the societal reaction.

Following Lemert (1951), the original theory distinguished between primary deviance, such as the hallucinations and thought disorder that are taken to be symptoms of schizophrenia, and those same behaviors as they occur in a person who is aware of his or her label as being mentally ill. The theory proposed that much primary deviance is of short duration or of little significance in the life of the bearer. But when people become aware of their label, they may come to play the role of the mentally ill, at first inadvertently, but later, perhaps, involuntarily. In other words, a group of symptoms may be stabilized, through self-consciousness and reaffirmation by others, as a "career" of mental illness.

The original theory, however, was insufficiently detailed. First, it was formulated in terms of abstract concepts, "black boxes," that were not clearly defined, like most other general theories of human behavior. Second, the causal links between these concepts were not specified. The theory described the societal reaction as a system without defining the major subsystems or the links between them. My final criticism is substantive, pointing toward a major deficit at the core of labeling theory: its omission of emotions. Although Goffman (1963) and others discussed stigma, they paid too little attention to emotions, particularly the emotion of shame.[1]

The original labeling theory was also oriented toward the formal labeling process, court hearings, and psychiatric examinations. Labeling (and nonlabeling) in these contexts was crude and overt. But in the family, as we argue here, labeling is covert. It depends upon innuendo, manner, unstated implications, and especially emotion. To detect it, one must interpret words and actions *in context.*

At this stage of theory development, reliable methods may be premature since they strip away context. The next step in developing a theory may be to understand a single case very well. Part/whole analysis allows one to show the relationship between the smallest parts of discourse and the very largest social system (Scheff 1990; 1997). When one can demonstrate an understanding of the relation between parts and wholes in a series of cases, the stage is then set for a research mode oriented toward testing hypotheses. Since mental illness at this point is still a mystery and a labyrinth, we need to generate models that are interesting enough to warrant testing—ones that have face validity.

This chapter outlines a theory and method that specify the role of unacknowledged shame in mental illness and in the societal reaction. The theory involves a model of feeling traps, recursive loops of shame and anger. The method involves the systematic interpretation of sequences of events in discourse. Discourse from a psychotherapy session is used to illustrate the theory, to allow us to envision the hypothesized moment-by-moment causal sequence.

PRIDE, SHAME, AND THE SOCIAL BOND

Cooley (1922) implied that pride and shame serve as intense and automatic bodily signs of the state of a system that is otherwise difficult to observe. Pride is the sign of an intact social bond; shame is the sign of a threatened one. The clearest outer marker of pride is holding up one's head in public, looking others in the eye, but indicating respect by alternately looking and looking away. In *overt* shame, one shrinks, averting or lowering one's gaze, casting only furtive glances at the other. In *bypassed* shame, one stares, outfacing the other.

Pride and shame thus serve as instinctive signals, both to the self and to the other, that communicate the state of the bond. By the state of the bond I mean the mix of solidarity and alienation in a particular social relationship. A completely secure bond would involve mutual understanding and mutual identification. A disrupted bond would involve no mutual understanding and no mutual identification. Most actual relationships fall somewhere between the two extremes. We react automatically to affirmations of and threats to bonds. But in early childhood most of us learn to disguise and ignore these signals. The idea of the social bond is repressed in modern societies, masked by the ideology of individualism. The emotions that express the bond—pride and shame—are also deeply repressed (Scheff 1990; Lewis 1971).

Lewis's (1971) work is particularly relevant to the conjecture under discussion. She found that in contexts high in potential for shame (as when a patient appears to suspect that the therapist is critical or judgmental), nonverbal indications of shame are plentiful. These include long or filled pauses ("well," "you know," "uh-uh-uh," and the like), repetition or self-interruption, and particularly, a lowering of the voice, often to the point of inaudibility. These markers are all suggestive of hiding behavior .

In these contexts, however, the painful affect of overt shame was virtually never acknowledged by name. Instead, other words were used, which Lewis interpreted to be a code language. *Insecure, awkward,* and *uncomfortable* are several examples from a long list. This language is analogous to the code language for designating other unmentionables, such as sexual or "toilet" terms. Like baby talk about body functions used with children, the denial of shame is institutionalized in the adult language of modern societies. Lewis's findings, like the approaches of Cooley, Goffman, and especially Elias (1978; 1982), suggest that shame is repressed in our civilization.

Although Goffman's, Elias's, and Lewis's treatments of shame are an advance over Cooley's in one way, in another way they are retrograde. Their treatment is much more specialized and detailed than Cooley's, whose discussion of the "self-regarding sentiments" is casual and brief. But Cooley had a vision of the whole system lacking in the more recent discussions. His treatment construes pride and shame to be polar opposites. It therefore lays the basis for our construct of the social bond; pride and shame are continuous signals of the state of the bond, an instant read-out of the "temperature" of the relationship.

The emotion of pride is absent from Goffman's and Lewis's formulations. Goffman's omission of pride is particularly disastrous. Since Lewis dealt only with psychotherapy discourse, we are free to imagine from her work that in normal conversation there is more pride than shame. But Goffman's treatments of "impression management," "face," and embarrassment concerned normal discourse, leaving the reader with the impression that all human activity is awash in a sea of shame. He nowhere envisioned a secure social bond, much less a well-ordered society built upon secure bonds. Goffman's omission of pride and secure bonds is particularly misleading for the study of deviance; it undercuts a crucial distinction between "normal" persons and labeled persons. Social situations usually generate pride for the former and shame for the latter. This difference has extraordinary consequences for the social system.

Goffman's (1963) treatment of stigma, although perceptive and useful, is not complete. Like other labeling theorists, his discussion is specialized, focusing on the behavioral aspects of stigma. He acknowledged the emotional component of the societal reaction only in passing. In particular, he mentioned shame only twice, once early in the essay: "[For the deviant] shame becomes a central possibility," (p. 7), and again at the end: "Once the dynamics of shameful differences are seen as a general feature of social life . . ." (p. 140).

Goffman frequently referred to shame or shame-related affects, but only indirectly ["self-hate and self-derogation" (p. 7)]. Without a working concept of the relationship between emotion and behavior, Goffman and the other stigma theorists were unable to show its central role in mental illness and the societal reaction. As a step toward this end, it is first necessary to review how emotions may cause protracted conflict.

An earlier report (Scheff 1987) described emotional bases of interminable conflicts. Like Watzlawick, Beavin, and Jackson (1967), I argue that some conflicts are unending; any particular quarrel within such conflicts is only a link in a continuing chain. Both primary and secondary deviance arises out of interminable conflicts. What is the cause of this type of conflict?

Lewis (1971; 1976; 1981a; 1981b) proposed that when shame is evoked but not acknowledged, an impasse occurs that has both social and psychological components. Here I sketch a model of impasse, a *triple spiral* of shame and rage *between* and *within* interactants. When persons have emotional reactions to their own emotions and to those of the other party, both become caught in a "feeling trap" (Lewis 1971) from which they cannot extricate themselves. The idea that emotions are contagious *between* individuals is familiar; the concept of spirals subsumes contagion both between and within parties to a conflict.

A NEW LABELING THEORY

My model follows from Lewis's (1971) analysis of therapy transcripts: shame is pervasive in clinical interaction, but it is invisible to interactants (and to researchers), unless Lewis's approach is used. [For methods that parallel Lewis's, see Gottschalk, Wingert, and Glaser's (1969) "shame-anxiety scale."]

Lewis (1971) referred to the internal shame-rage process as a "feeling trap," as "anger bound by shame," or "humiliated fury." Kohut's (1971) concept, "narcissistic rage," appears to be the same affect, since he viewed it as a compound of shame and rage. When one is angry that one is ashamed, or ashamed that one is angry, then one might be ashamed to be so upset over something so "trivial." Such anger and shame are rarely acknowledged and are difficult to detect and to dispel. Shame-rage spirals may be brief, lasting a matter of minutes, or they can last for hours, days, or a lifetime, as bitter hatred or resentment.

Brief sequences of shame-rage may be quite common. Escalation is avoided through withdrawal, conciliation, or some other tactic. In this chapter a less common type of conflict is described. Watzlawick et al. (1967, pp. 107–108) called it "symmetrical escalation." Since such conflicts have no limits, they may be lethal. I describe the cognitive and emotional components of symmetrical escalation, as far as they are evidenced in the transcript.

LABELING IN THE FAMILY: A CASE STUDY
(Based on Scheff 1989)

Labov and Fanshel (1977) conducted an exhaustive microanalysis of a large segment of a psychotherapy session. They analyzed not only what was said but also how it was said, interpreting both words and manner (the paralanguage). They based their interpretations upon microscopic details of paralanguage, such as pitch and loudness contours. Words and paralanguage are used to infer inner states: intentions, feelings, and meanings.

With such attention to detail, Labov and Fanshel were able to convey un-stated *implications*. Their report is evocative; one forms vivid pictures of pa-tient and therapist and of their relationship. One can also infer aspects of the relationship between Rhoda and her family, since Rhoda reports family dia-logues. Labov and Fanshel showed that the dispute style in Rhoda's family is indirect: conflict is generated by nonverbal means and by implication.

Indirect inferences, from a dialogue that is only reported, are made in order to construct a causal model. Obviously, in future research they will need to be validated by observations of actual family dialogue. It is reassuring, how-ever, to find that many aspects of her own behavior that Rhoda reports as occurring in the dialogues with her family are directly observable in her di-alogue with the therapist. For example, the absence of greeting, and Rhoda's covert aggression in the dialogue she reports with her aunt can be observed directly in the session itself (not included in this chapter but discussed in Scheff 1989).

The Feud between Rhoda and Her Family

Rhoda was a nineteen-year-old college student who had a prior diagnosis of anorexia. She had been hospitalized because of her rapid weight loss, from 140 to 70 pounds. When her therapy began, she weighed 90 pounds. At five feet five inches in height, she was dangerously underweight.

Her therapy sessions took place in New York City in the 1960s. Rhoda lived with her mother and her aunt, Editha; her married sister also figures in the di-alogue. The session that was analyzed by Labov and Fanshel was the twenty-fifth in a longer series, which appeared to end successfully. The therapist re-ported improvement at termination. At a five-year follow-up, Rhoda was of normal weight, married, and raising her own children.

Labov and Fanshel focused on the web of conflict in Rhoda's life, mainly with her family and to a lesser extent with her therapist. The conflict was not open but hidden. The authors showed that Rhoda's statements (and those she attributed to the members of her family) were packed with innuendo. They inferred that the style of dispute in Rhoda's family was indirect: although the family members were aggressive toward each other and hurt by each other, both their aggression and their hurt were denied.

Labov and Fanshel's method was to state explicitly as verbal propositions what was only implied in the actual dialogue. This method proposed a cog-nitive structure for the conflict in Rhoda's family: it translated utterances, words, and paralanguage into purely verbal statements. The set of verbal statements served as a compact, clarifying blueprint for a dense tissue of complex ma-neuvers that were otherwise difficult to detect and understand.

In addition to this type of analysis, Labov and Fanshel also used another. Following the lead of the therapist, they pointed out cues that were indicative of unacknowledged anger. To reveal this emotion, they used verbal and nonverbal signs: words and paralanguage (such as pitch and loudness). Hidden challenges in Rhoda's family were made in anger and resulted in anger. Rhoda's therapist made explicit reference to this matter: "So there's a lot of anger passing back and forth" (5.27[c]; the numbers refer to the Rhoda transcript, Labov and Fanshel 1977, pp. 363–371). There were also myriad indications of unacknowledged anger and other emotions in the session itself.

Emotions were not central to Labov and Fanshel's study, but they are to mine. Building upon their assessment of cognitive conflict, and their (and the therapist's) analysis of anger, I show shame sequences in the session that were apparently unnoticed by both patient and therapist. Labov and Fanshel frequently noted the presence of embarrassment and of the combined affect they called "helpless anger," but they made little use of these events.

My study leads me to conclude that labeling occurs at two different levels—the informal and the formal. At the informal level, labeling is quite symmetrical: Rhoda labeled and blamed Aunt Editha and her mother just as much as they labeled and blamed her. The family members casually insulted each other almost constantly. In some sentences, several different insults were implied at once. As Labov and Fanshel pointed out, conflict seemed to be endemic in this family.

At the formal level of labeling, however, there was no symmetry whatsoever. Although the mother and the aunt were just as violent with their insults, threats, and rejections as Rhoda, it was only Rhoda who was physically violent; she tried to starve herself. In contrast to the constant verbal violence, Rhoda's overt violence was highly visible; her dangerously low body weight bore ostensible witness to her self-assault. Although the verbal violence seemed to be visible to the therapist and was documented by Labov and Fanshel, it was invisible in Rhoda's community. If labeling theory is going to lead to further understanding of mental illness, it will need to take a new direction, to make visible what has hitherto been invisible; violence in the microworld of moment-to-moment social interaction.

I use two excerpts (Labov and Fanshel 1977, pp. 364, 365). The first involves Rhoda's relationship with her mother; the second, with her Aunt Editha. The first excerpt occurred early in the session—it deals with a telephone conversation that Rhoda reported. The mother was temporarily staying at the house of Rhoda's sister, Phyllis. (Since pauses were significant in their analysis, Labov and Fanshel signified their length: each period equals .3 second.)

Excerpt 1

1.8 R.: An-nd so—when—I called her t'day, I said, "Well, when do you plan t'come *home*?"

1.9 R.: So she said, "Oh, why!"

1.10 R.: An-nd I said, "Well, things are getting just a little too *much*! [laugh] This is—it's jis' getting too hard, and . . . I—"

1.11 R.: She s'd t'me, "Well, why don't you tell *Phyllis* that!"

1.12 R.: So I said, "Well, I haven't talked to her lately."

Rhoda, a full-time student, argues that she can't keep house without help. Her mother puts her off by referring her to Phyllis. The implication—that the mother is there at Phyllis's behest—is not explored by the therapist. Rather, she asks Rhoda about getting help from Aunt Editha. Rhoda's response:

Excerpt 2

2.6[a]R.: I said t'her (breath) w-one time—I asked her—I said t'her.

[b]: "Wellyouknow, wdy'mind takin' thedustrag an'justdust around?"

2.7R.: Sh's's, "Oh-I-I—it looks clean to me," . . .

2.8[a]R.: An' then I went like *this*.

[b]: an' I said to her, "*That* looks *clean* t'you?"

(It appears that at this point, Rhoda had drawn her finger across a dusty surface and thrust her dusty finger into Editha's face.)

2.9[a]R.: And she sort of. . . . *I* d'no—sh'sort of gave me a funny look as if I—hurt her in some way,

[b]: and I mean I didn' *mean* to, I didn' *yell* and *scream*.

[c]: All I did to her was that "*That* looks clean to you?" . . .

The therapist persists that Rhoda may be able to obtain help from Editha. In a later segment (not shown), Rhoda denies this possibility.

Rhoda's Helpless Anger toward Her Aunt

I will begin analysis with the least complex segment, the dialogue that Rhoda reports between herself and her aunt (2.5–2.9). Labov and Fanshel (1977) showed a thread of underlying anger, anger that is denied by both parties.

Rhoda has explained prior to this excerpt that dust "bothers" her—that is, makes her angry. The authors argue that the request that Editha "dust around" (2.6[b]) involves an angry challenge to Editha's authority, a challenge that neither side acknowledges. It assumes that the house is dusty, that Editha knows it, that she has ignored her obligation to do something about it, and that Rhoda has the right to remind her of it. Although Rhoda uses "mitigating" devices, speaking rapidly and casually, she ignores the etiquette that would have avoided challenge.

[Labov and Fanshel wrote, "The making of requests is a delicate business and requires a great deal of supporting ritual to avoid damaging personal relations surrounding it" (1977, p. 96).] To avoid challenge, Rhoda might have begun with an apology and explanation: *"You know, Aunt Editha, this is a busy time for me, I need your help so I can keep up with my schoolwork." Rhoda's actual request is abrupt.

Editha's response is also abrupt: "Oh-I-I—it looks clean to me . . . " She has refused Rhoda's request, intimating inaccuracy in Rhoda's appraisal. The ritual necessary to refuse a request without challenge is at least as elaborate as that of making one. Editha could have shown Rhoda deference: *"I'm sorry Rhoda, but . . . ," followed by an explanation of why she was not going to honor the request.

Rhoda's response to what she appears to have taken as an insult is brief and emphatic: She contemptuously dismisses Editha's contention. She wipes her finger across a dusty surface and thrusts it close to Editha's face: "*That* looks *clean* to you?" Labov and Fanshel noted the aggressive manner in Rhoda's rebuttal: she stresses the words *that* and *clean,* as if Editha were a child or hard of hearing. They identified the pattern of pitch and loudness as the "Yiddish rise-fall intonation": *"By *you* that's a *monkey* wrench?" implying repudiation of the other's point of view. "If you think this is clean, you're crazy" (p. 202). Rhoda's response escalates the level of conflict: she has openly challenged Editha's competence.

Finally, Rhoda describes Editha's response, which is not verbal but gestural: she gives Rhoda a "funny look as if I—hurt her in some way." Rhoda denies any intention of hurting Editha, and that Editha has any grounds for being hurt: "I didn't yell and scream," implying that Editha is unreasonable.

Labov and Fanshel noted the presence of anger not only in the original interchange but also in Rhoda's retelling of it. The nonverbal signs, they said— choking, hesitation, glottalization, and whine—are indications of *helpless anger*: Rhoda "is so choked with emotion at the unreasonableness of Editha's behavior that she can not begin to describe it accurately" (ibid., p. 191). Helpless anger, the authors wrote, characterizes Rhoda's statements *throughout the whole session:* "she finds herself unable to cope with behavior of others that injures her and seems to her unreasonable" (ibid.).

Labov and Fanshel further noted that her expressions of helpless anger were "mitigated":

> All of these expressions of emotion are counterbalanced with mitigating expressions indicating that Rhoda's anger is not extreme and that she is actually taking a moderate, adult position on the question of cleanliness. Thus she is not angered by the situation, it only "bothers" her. Even this is too strong; Rhoda further mitigates the expression to "sort of bothers me." (ibid.)

Mitigation in this instance means denial: Rhoda denies her anger by disguising it with euphemisms.

What is the source of all the anger and denial? Let us start with Rhoda's helpless anger during her report of the dialogue. Helpless anger, according to Lewis (1971), is a variant of shame-anger: we are ashamed of our helplessness. In retelling the story, Rhoda is caught up in a shame-anger sequence: shame that she feels rejected by Editha, anger at Editha, shame at her anger, and so on.

Helpless anger has been noted by others besides Lewis and Kohut. Nietzsche ([1887] 1967) referred to a similar affect ("impotent rage") as the basis for resentment. Scheler ([1912] 1961) used Nietzsche's idea in his study of *ressentiment*—pathological resentment. Horowitz (1981), finally, dealt with a facet of helpless anger under the heading "self-righteous anger."

Rhoda and her family are caught in a web of *ressentiment,* to use Scheler's term. Each side attributes the entire blame to the other; neither side sees its own contribution. As Labov and Fanshel showed, one of Rhoda's premises is that *she* is reasonable, and the members of her family are unreasonable. The reported dialogues with her family imply that the family holds the opposite premise: that *they* are reasonable, but she is unreasonable.

My theory suggests that the dialogue between Rhoda and Editha is only a segment of a continuous quarrel. Since it is ongoing, it may not be possible to locate a particular beginning; any event recovered is only a link in a chain (Watzlawick et al. 1967, p. 58). Starting at an arbitrary point, suppose that Rhoda is "hurt" by Editha's failure to help. That is, she feels rejected, shamed by Editha's indifference, and angry at Editha for this reason. She is also ashamed of being angry, however. Her anger is bound by shame. For this reason it cannot be acknowledged, let alone discharged. Editha may be in a similar trap. Rhoda is irritable and disrespectful, which could cause Editha shame and anger. She could experience Rhoda's hostility as rejecting, arousing her own feelings of helpless anger. Reciprocating chains of shame and anger on both sides cause symmetrical escalation.

The Impasse between Rhoda and Her Mother

Excerpt 1, as reported by Rhoda, may point to the core conflict. It is brief—only three complete exchanges—but as Labov and Fanshel showed, it is packed with innuendo. My analysis follows theirs, but expands it to include emotion dynamics.

Rhoda's first line, as she reports the conversation, is seemingly innocuous: "Well, when do you plan t'come home?" To reveal the unstated implications, Labov and Fanshel (1977) analyzed understandings about role obligations in Rhoda's family. Rhoda's statement is a demand for action, disguised as a question. They pointed out affective elements: it contains sarcasm (p. 156), criticism (p. 161), challenge (pp. 157, 159), and rudeness (p. 157). The challenge and criticism are inherent in a demand from a child that implies that the mother is neglecting her obligations.

Implicit in their comments is the point I made about Rhoda's approach to her aunt. It was possible for Rhoda to have requested action without insult, by showing deference, reaffirming the mother's status, and providing an explanation and apology. Rhoda's request is rude because it contains none of these elements.

Rhoda's habitual rudeness is also indicated by the absence of two ceremonial forms from all her dialogues, not only with her family, but also with her therapist: any form of greeting, and the use of the other's name and title. Does Rhoda merely forget these elements in her report of the dialogues? Not likely, since they are also missing in the session itself. Labov and Fanshel tell us that the transcript begins "with the very first words spoken in the session; there is no small talk or preliminary settling down. . . . Instead the patient herself immediately begins the discussion." Rhoda neglects to greet the therapist or call her by name. Since Rhoda is junior to the therapist, her aunt, and her mother, the absence of greeting, name, and title is a mark of inadequate deference toward persons of higher status. Rhoda's casual manner is rude.

The mother's response is just as rude and just as indirect. According to Rhoda's report, her mother also neglects greetings and the use of names. Like Rhoda's aunt, she neither honors the request nor employs the forms necessary to avoid giving offense. Rather than answering Rhoda's question, she asks another question—a delay that is the first step in rejecting the request.

Labov and Fanshel stated that the intonation contour of the mother's response ("Oh, *why*'") suggests "heavy implication." They inferred: *"I told you so; many, many, times I have told you so." [When Rhoda gives a second account of this dialogue (4.12–4.15), she reports that the mother actually said, "See, I told you so."] What is it that the mother, and presumably others, has told Rhoda many times? The answer to this question may be at the core of the quarrel between Rhoda and her family.

Whether it is only an implication or an actual statement, the mother's I-told-you-so escalates the conflict from the specific issue at hand— whether she is going to come home—to a more general level: Rhoda's status. Rhoda's offensiveness in her opening question involves her mother's status only at this moment. The mother's response involves a general issue. Is Rhoda a responsible and therefore a worthwhile person, or is she sick, mad, or irresponsible?

Labeling, Shame, and Insecure Bonds

At a superficial level, the mother's I-told-you-so statement involves only Rhoda's ability to function on her own. As can be seen from Rhoda's complaints at the end of the session, however, this implication is symbolic of a larger set of accusations that Rhoda sees her mother and sister as leveling at her: she is either willfully or crazily not taking care of herself, starving herself, and she doesn't care about the effect of her behavior on her family. Her family's basic accusation, Rhoda feels, is that she is upsetting them, but she doesn't care. Rhoda formulates this accusation at the end of the transcript.

Excerpt 3

> **T.:** What are they feeling?
>
> **5.26R.:** . . . that I'm doing it on purp—like, I w's—like they . . . well-they s-came out an'tol' me in so many words that they worry and worry an' I seem to take this very lightly.

To Rhoda, the mother's I-told-you-so epitomizes a host of infuriating, shaming charges about her sanity, responsibility, and lack of consideration. Note particularly that the labeling process to which Rhoda refers here is not explicit; it occurs through innuendo.

The labeling of Rhoda by the other family members and its emotional consequences underlie the whole family conflict. Yet it can be detected only by a subtle process of inference, understanding the meaning of words and gestures in context, in actual discourse. Both the theory and the method of the original labeling theory were too abstract to detect this basic process.

Rhoda responds (in 1.10) not to the underlying implication of her mother's evasion but to the surface question, "Why do you want to know?" Because, she answers, " . . . things are getting just a little too much . . . " The key element in Rhoda's response is the *affect*. Labov and Fanshel stated that the paralanguage [choked laughter, hesitation, glottalization, and long silence (p. 170)] is an indication of embarrassment (p. 171). Rhoda responds to her mother's accusations by becoming *ashamed*. The shame sequence that is described is a marker for stigmatization that is otherwise hidden behind polite words.

Rhoda's shame may indicate that she feels that her family's charges have some basis, or that the implied rejection leads her to feel worthless, or both. Since no anger is visible at this instant, it is either absent or bypassed. The verbal text, however, suggests that Rhoda is feeling shame and guilt. She is acknowledging that she needs her mother—a need she has repeatedly denied in the past. She may feel that she is at fault for this reason.

Labov and Fanshel contrasted the force of the mother's response with the weakness of Rhoda's comment (at 1.10). The mother says, "Why don't you tell Phyllis that?" Labov and Fanshel stated that the hesitation and embarrassment that characterize 1.10 are absent from this response. It is a forceful rejection of Rhoda's claims and, by implication, a criticism of Rhoda for even making the request. The mother's emotional response to Rhoda's embarrassment is not simply unsympathetic; it is aggressively rejecting. From the emotional standpoint, Rhoda's back is to the wall. She is trapped in the helpless role of the blamed, with her mother as the aggressive blamer.

The analysis of shame in this dialogue points to an otherwise hidden issue.

At this moment we can see that in her family, Rhoda has literally no one to whom she can turn. She is at odds with her aunt. We know from her reports of her sister's comments that Rhoda and she are also in a tangle. No father is mentioned. Rhoda and her family are in a perpetual war, a war hidden beneath the surface of conventional discourse. All of Rhoda's bonds are threatened, yet she has no way of understanding her complete alienation.

The stage is set for violent emotion and/or violent behavior: for mental illness (Rhoda appears to be delusional about her eating and body weight), murder, or suicide (in this case, self-starvation). That the potential for suicide arises when individuals have no one to whom they can turn was conjectured by Sacks (1966) on the basis of his analysis of calls to a suicide prevention center. The repression of shame and the bondlessness that is its cause and effect can give rise to primary deviance in the form of mental illness, murder, or suicide.

In Rhoda's response (1.12), she continues in the role of the one at fault: "Well, I haven't talked to her lately." Her mother has defeated her on all counts. She has refused Rhoda's request without the ritual that would protect Rhoda's "face"; she has implied a victory over Rhoda ("I told you so") that undercuts Rhoda's status, and she has criticized her for making an inappropriate request to the wrong person.

Rhoda appears to feel too baffled, upset, and helpless for an angry counterattack. Her anger at her mother may feel too shameful to countenance. It is reserved for lesser targets: her aunt, her sister, and the therapist. Her mother's rejection, with the implied threat of abandonment, could be the basic source of Rhoda's shame.

Even to the casual reader, the mother's tactics are transparent. Why is Rhoda so baffled by them? Why didn't she use a response like the one suggested by the authors: *"Oh, come off it, Ma! You know it's really up to you when you come home, not Phyllis. Get off my case!"

Rhoda's ineptness may be due to her intense shame, evoked beginning with the first question, asking her mother for help. In this instance the massiveness of the unacknowledged shame is befuddling almost to the point of paralysis.

In the overt form of shame, one is so flustered that speech is disrupted, with inaudibility, repetition, stuttering, and fragmentation. Even though she is only reporting the dialogue, Rhoda's speech shows many of these markers. Bypassed shame, on the other hand, may disrupt one's ability to think clearly, forcing one into a holding pattern, repeating set responses not particularly appropriate to the moment (Scheff 1987). This dialogue suggests that Rhoda is overwhelmed with both kinds of shame.

At the heart of the quarrel is a series of threats between Rhoda and her mother. As in all interminable quarrels, it is not possible to identify the first link. I begin with Rhoda's basic threat, without signifying that it came first:

*"If you don't stop shaming me, I will starve myself!" Her mother's basic threat: *"If you don't stop shaming me, I'll abandon you!"

The abandonment threat in this case is literal: the mother has left Rhoda to stay with her other daughter. Normally, the threat of abandonment would be largely symbolic; carrying out a threat of abandonment is probably rare. But whether it is real or symbolic, threats of abandonment may be the key link in the causal chain.

This chain has potentially lethal force because none of it is visible to both participants. There are four links: (1) Rhoda's shame in response to her mother's behavior toward her; (2) her threat to starve; (3) the mother's shame in response to Rhoda's behavior; (4) her threat to abandon Rhoda. Rhoda is aware of none of these links. Nearest to her awareness is the mother's threat to abandon her, and next the shaming by her mother. Rhoda is unaware that her mother is shamed by Rhoda's aggressive and self-destructive behavior, and she denies that she is starving herself. The mother is aware of only one link: Rhoda's threat to starve herself. Because of this awareness, she talks to and about Rhoda in code, not daring to mention Rhoda's threat. Her shame over Rhoda's behavior, her own shaming of Rhoda, and her threat to abandon Rhoda apparently are not experienced by her.

The driving force in the quarrel is not the anger that was interpreted by the therapist but the shame in the field between Rhoda and her family. The anger in this family is both generated and bound by shame. Rhoda experiences her mother's threat of abandonment and her mother's anger as shaming. The mother experiences Rhoda's threat of self-starvation and Rhoda's anger as shaming. The symmetry is complete: each side is threatened and shamed by the other, and each side can see only the other's threat.

The system of threats and hidden emotions is comparable to that preceding conflict between nations (Scheff 1994). Each side feels its credibility would be diminished by backing down in the face of threat. Each side therefore escalates the level of threat. The resulting emotions have no limit, unless outside mediation occurs or shame is dispelled. "War fever" may be code language for collective shame-rage spirals.

The theory advanced here attempts to explain the emotional sources of mental illness, and the excessive force of the societal reaction to mental illness, the roots of primary and secondary deviance. Rhoda and her family are caught in an interminable conflict that is driven by triple spirals of shame and anger within and between the disputants. For brevity, I have not included my (1989) analysis of the transaction between Rhoda and her therapist, but because of its relevance to the argument, I provide a brief summary.

Although Rhoda attacks the therapist surreptitiously, using the same tactics she uses against the authority figures in her family—her mother and her aunt—the therapist is too wily to become enmeshed in them. She gets angry, but she doesn't attack Rhoda back, as Rhoda's mother and aunt do. By avoiding enmeshment in the family conflict, the therapist is able to form a secure bond with Rhoda, leading ultimately to a successful course of therapy.

Research in the labeling tradition suggests that therapists like this one are probably rare. Therapists and other agents outside the family often become enmeshed in family conflicts, usually aiding with the family against the patient. Bowen's (1978) seminal analysis of family systems implies this course. Several of our earlier case studies illustrate the enmeshment of the outside agents on the side of the family (Retzinger 1989; Scheff 1966; 1987).

LABELING BY PSYCHIATRISTS

Retzinger's study (1989) of a psychiatric interview goes further; she shows how the psychiatrist is enmeshed with the family position and how this enmeshment leads to renewed psychiatric symptoms, as predicted by Lewis's theory (1981a,b). The theory proposed here explains the extraordinary forces underlying mental illness and the reaction to it, chain reactions of shame and anger, feelings traps both in patients and in those reacting to them.

A recent study of mental illness using a strictly biographical method has produced findings parallel to ours. Porter (1990) provides an even-handed assessment of endogenous and environmental contributions to the mental illness of a large number of well-documented cases. His summary of the findings for one case—the nineteenth-century patient John Perceval—can be taken to represent his conclusions for the majority of his cases:

> Perceval believed that religious terror had brought on his insanity, and that the behavior of his family had exacerbated it. But *the real cause of the appalling severity and prolongation of his condition was the medico-psychiatric treatment* he had received. Perceval unambiguously condemned as intrinsically counter-productive the very philosophy of placing mad people in lunatic asylums. It set the lunatic amongst "strangers" precisely when he *needed to be with his fellows* in familiar surroundings. It estranged him from his family. It put him in the charge of an unknown doctor, rather than those members of the caring professions he knew well, his regular physician or his clergyman. It set him in the midst of fellow lunatics, who, if truly mad, must surely be those people least capable of sustaining the mind of one who had just been crushed under a terrible blow. Precisely at the moment when a person needed his morale to be boosted, he was thrown into a situation that must *"degrade him in his own estimation."* (pp. 180–181, emphasis added)

This statement clearly supports labeling theory and points particularly to the two elements in labeling that are emphasized by the new theory: the weakening of social bonds and the accompanying unacknowledged shame. That the psychiatric treatments of the composer Robert Schumann and the dancer Nijinsky resulted in the complete severing of their social bonds is particularly shocking (Porter 1990, pp. 65–71, 71–75).

The position that Porter, a historian, takes toward his findings seems equivocal. He cites none of the labeling theory literature; he states that he sides neither with the patients nor with the psychiatrists. Yet his closing message acknowledges some strain. The first line of his conclusion reads, "This book has not pleaded a cause" (p. 231). He goes on to say that his aim has been merely to focus attention on a body of forgotten writings, the memoirs of the mad. Yet at the end of the conclusion, he states, "[C]learly, no reader will have taken the opening statement of this Conclusion at face value" (p. 232). For reasons that are never stated, Porter is reluctant to acknowledge the implications of his findings. He seems to make the error of equating taking a stand on his own findings with "pleading a cause."

CONCLUSION

The case in this chapter contains the three elements fundamental to my theory: inadequate bonds, dysfunctional communication, and destructive conflict. Before her contact with the therapist, Rhoda appears to have been alienated from everyone in her family. No father is mentioned, and she seems to have the barest cognitive attunement with her mother and aunt and virtually no understanding at the emotional level.

The dialogues with her mother and aunt that Rhoda reports clearly indicate dysfunctional patterns of communication. She and her mother are extremely indirect, evasive, and withholding with each other, and she and her aunt are violently disrespectful, although in underhanded ways. It is of great interest that although she tries the same tactics she used in her family on the therapist, the therapist is able to sidestep them, giving Rhoda what turns out to be important lessons in how to communicate directly but respectfully.

The theme of violence is present in these dialogues only in the form of Rhoda's attempts at self-starvation. Like virtually all the other important issues in Rhoda's family, these attempts are disguised and denied: Rhoda claims that she is only dieting and that she is not underweight. As in most important issues in social communication, contextual, prospective, and retrospective knowledge beyond the discourse itself is needed to interpret the meaning of statements and events.

Support for the theory is also found in the cues for hidden emotion that both the therapist and Labov and Fanshel point out in their interpretations. Although the therapist only interprets Rhoda's and her family's anger, Labov and Fanshel's careful analysis of microscopic cues in verbal and nonverbal behavior provides support for our theory of shame-rage spirals. Their analysis frequently pointed to instances of "embarrassment" (shame) and "helpless anger" (shame-anger), suggesting the sequences required by the theory. The theory of shame-rage spirals fills in the wiring diagram of the black boxes in labeling theory: unacknowledged alienation and shame drive the labeling machine.

As in its earlier formulation, our extended labeling theory implies a critique of conventional psychiatry, which is individualistic and affirms the status quo. In focusing exclusively on Rhoda's pathology, it denies the pathology in the family system of which she is a part and, by implication, in the larger social system, our current civilization.

The next step in following up the theory and method developed here would be a systematic comparative study of labeling and nonlabeling in actual families (rather than conversations reported by the patient in the Rhoda study) and outside the family, in schools, jobs, and psychiatric examinations. Unifying case study and comparative methods, as I am suggesting here, is a return to the morphological method used in the development of the science of biology, rather than the specialization and compartmentalization of theory and method current in the social sciences.

NOTE

1. Peggy Thoits and John Braithwaite are exceptions. Thoits has published a study (1985) that connects emotions and labeling, and Braithwaite (1989) a theory of stigmatization that explicitly links stigma and shame. Braithwaite's framework links low crime rates with "reintegrative" or what we would call normal shame, and high crime rates with stigmatization (or recursive shame). He also makes a connection between normal shame and community. His work implies the fundamental link between shame and the social bond described here.

V

SUMMARY AND REVIEW

10

Conclusion

This final chapter recapitulates the earlier discussion and adds three final suggestions: a recommendation concerning interpretation of psychiatric symptoms (and its implications for research on mental illness), a theoretical formulation in which the investigation of the causes of mental illness is translated into a study of the dynamics of status *systems,* and recommendations for research and treatment involving the emotional/relational world.

The theory of mental illness outlined in the earlier chapters is that the symptoms of mental illness can be considered to be violations of residual social norms, and that the careers of residual deviants can most effectively be considered as dependent on the societal reaction and the processes of role-playing, when role-playing is viewed as part of a social rather than an exclusively individual system.

The theoretical formulation of symptoms as normative violations places great stress on the social context in which symptomatic behavior occurs as do the findings concerning the nearly automatic procedures in psychiatric screening. Implied in these considerations is a relationship among symptoms, context, and meaning that may be important in future research.

SYMPTOM, CONTEXT, AND MEANING

The two studies of the societal reaction to mental illness published in the first two editions of this book (Scheff 1966; 1984) showed that involuntary confinement in mental hospitals, in the jurisdictions studied, seemed largely based on the presumption of illness by officials. Because these studies were conducted over thirty years ago, and because of substantial changes in mental health laws, I have not republished them in this edition. Is this presumption intrinsic to systems that seek to control mental disorder?

The officials whom we interviewed at the time felt that in virtually every case, the family or other complainants sought hospitalization only after exhausting all other alternatives. According to these officials, complainants seek hospitalization only when driven to it by the repeated, meaningless, and uncontrollable behavior of the prospective patient. Prior studies provide support for the belief that some families bend over backwards to avoid hospitalization. Yarrow and others (1955) have shown that the defining of repeated rule breaking as a psychiatric problem is avoided for rather long periods of time.

The officials, then, conceived of the families and other complainants as very reluctant to even consider hospitalization except in cases in which its necessity was a forgone conclusion. Except for some of the court clerks, the officials did not seem to consider the possibility that some of the complainants might have taken action too quickly rather than too slowly. Are there families in which there was "something wrong" less with the patient than with the family? In their study of scapegoating in the family, Vogel and Bell (1961) found that parental inadequacies and marital conflict were often projected onto the weakest child in the family, so that he was "induced" into the role of the deviant. Some empirical evidence for such "induced" roles in complaints about alleged mental illness was found in Philadelphia, where prehospitalization investigation showed that in some 25% of the complaints, it was the complainer, rather than the prospective patient, who was obviously suspect (Linden 1964).

The clearest example of the bias of the family's complaints is provided in the work of Laing and Esterson (1964). They present detailed discussions of persons diagnosed as schizophrenics, showing that what is represented to be psychotic symptoms is usually rebellion against extremely tyrannical or bizarre parents. Findings such as theirs have given rise to the belief among many researchers that it is often the families, rather than the patients, who are really "crazy," and that the symptoms of the patients are only normal reactions to very unusual situations.

The formulations concerning "family pathology," although they lead to a more adequate perspective, probably represent only a partial resolution. In his paper on the social dynamics of paranoia, Lemert (1962) points out that the complainants who initiate action against a nonconformer may be caught up, with the nonconformer, in a spiral of misinformation, incorrect attributions, and, ultimately, in delusions on both sides. According to Lemert's formulation, it is the internal political and social-psychological process of small groups that can lead to extrusion, first informally and later formally, from the group. Thus, the determinants of extrusion may lie not in pathology of the complainants but in the social-psychological situation in the host group, which may generate elementary collective behavior.

Lemert's paper also may serve as a corrective to the view that only the family setting can lead to the kind of nonconforming behavior that is labeled as mental illness. The small groups that Lemert discusses are not in families but in organizations: factions in businesses, factories, and schools. Obviously, however, the faction politics, selective perception, and the attenuation and breakdown of communication between the suspect individual and the rest of the group can occur in families in ways similar to those described by Lemert in large organizations.

Like Laing and Esterson, Lemert indicates that psychiatric symptoms can be understood if seen in the context of the family or group situation in which they occurred. The grave weakness of psychiatric decision-making is the absence of the situational elements. As one psychiatrist pointed out some time ago:

> A major source of difficulty in psychiatric diagnosis and evaluation is that symptoms are considered to be pathological manifestations *regardless of the context in which they appear. In themselves, however, symptoms are neither normal nor abnormal:* they derive significance only in relation to the [situation in which they occur]. (Coleman 1964; emphasis added)

The refraction that occurs because the context is omitted in psychiatric examinations is nicely documented by Laing and Esterson (1964). With symptom after symptom, they are able to point out how meaningful behavior, when taken out of context, is perceived to be a psychiatric symptom.

To take the first case they discuss, Maya, a 28-year-old mental patient, was diagnosed at 18 years of age as a paranoid schizophrenic, with various symptoms such as auditory hallucinations, ideas of reference and influence, and varying delusions of persecution. Through lengthy and detailed interviews with the patient and her parents, Laing and Esterson (1964) were able to put these symptoms in a very different light. By probing into an incident in which the auditory hallucinations were alleged to have occurred, the patient was led to these statements: "She said she had felt quite well at the time: she did not feel that it had to do with her illness. She was responsible for it. She had not been told to act like that by her voices. *The voices, she said, were her own thoughts, anyway*" (p. 25; emphasis added). With regard to the alleged ideas of influence, Laing and Esterson found over a year after they began to interview the family, that the father and mother had the idea that Maya could read their thoughts, and that they (the parents) had actually tested her "powers" with experiments in their home. Similarly, the ideas of reference were understandable in context:

An idea of reference that she had was that something she could not fathom was going on between her parents, seemingly about her. Indeed there was. When they were interviewed together, her mother and father kept exchanging with each other a constant series of nods, winks, gestures, knowing smiles, so obvious to the observer, that he commented on them after twenty minutes of the first such interview. They continued, however, unabated and denied. (p. 24)

It would appear, then, that the patient's ideas of reference and influence and delusions of persecution were merely descriptions of her parents' behavior toward her. Laing and Esterson document many such misinterpretations in all of the cases they studied.[1]

How do such glaring misinterpretations occur in psychiatric screening? One obvious cause is simple lack of information. Lemert worked for several years in collecting information about 8 cases from interviews with relatives, neighbors, physicians, employers, police, attorneys, and jury members. Laing and Esterson spent an average of 25 hours in interviewing each of the 11 families in their study, with a range of from 16 to 50 hours per family. It is obvious that the kind of contextual information that they uncovered could not be collected in an ideal psychiatric interview of 1 or 2 hours, much less in the psychiatric interviews we observed in a midwestern state, which took from 5 to 17 minutes.

One reason, then, that the behavior of alleged mental patients is thought to be meaningless is that the extremely brief and peremptory psychiatric and judicial interviews shear away most of the information about the context in which the "symptomatic" behavior occurred. There is another kind of factor that leads to the presumption of illness, however, which is more or less independent of the amount of time taken in screening. The medical model, in which nonconforming behavior tends to be seen as a symptom of "mental illness," leads in itself to the ignoring of context (Goffman 1959).

The concept of *disease,* as it is commonly understood, refers to a process that occurs within the body of an individual. Psychiatric symptoms, therefore, are conceived to be a part of a system of behavior that is located entirely within the patient and that is independent of the social context within which the "symptoms" occur.

It is almost a truism, however, among social psychologists and students of language that the meaning of behavior is not primarily a property of the behavior itself, but of the relation between the behavior and the context in which it occurs. In his paper, Garfinkel (1964) has shown how even the most routine and conventional behavior loses its meaning when the penumbra of subtle but multitudinous understandings is omitted. The medical model, since it is based on a conception of physical, rather than social events, fractures the figure-ground relationship between behavior and social context, leading almost inevitably to a bias of seeing suspect behavior as meaningless. Given such a bias, even very extensive and detailed psychiatric interviews would not guarantee against a presumption of illness.

This discussion suggests that both the theory and practice of psychiatric screening tend to be biased toward seeing behavior of the alleged mentally ill as meaningless, and therefore as symptomatic. The practice of screening, by its brevity, tends to omit contextual information, and the theory, based as it is on the medical model, tends to ignore the contextual information that is available. The remainder of this section is devoted to a brief discussion of some of the implications of these findings for theory and method in the field of abnormal psychology.

Perhaps the clearest implication is the gross unreliability of psychiatric diagnosis as an indication of anything about the behavior of the mental patient. The process of psychiatric screening would appear to be more sensitive to economic, political, and social-psychological pressures on the screening agents than to most aspects of the patient's behavior. This proposition suggests that a basic reorientation is needed in psychological theory and research concerning "mental illness." Too often psychologists and other social scientists simply accept the results of the psychiatric screening process as essentially valid. It is a great convenience to the researcher, after all, to accept society's ready-made measurement of that difficult and elusive dependent variable, psychiatric abnormality, so that he is free to make precise, reliable, and valid measurements of his favorite independent variables. Because of this acceptance, there is now an alarmingly large number of studies that present the ludicrous situation in which there is a refined and sophisticated handling of the independent variable, whether it be genetic, biochemical, psychological, cultural, or a host of others; the measurement of "mental illness," however, is left to the obscure, almost unknown, vagaries of the process of psychiatric screening.

The acceptance of society's official diagnosis is also convenient for the researcher, because it aligns him with the status quo, thus avoiding almost certain conflict with the agencies (such as the hospitals and courts) whose cooperation he needs in order to carry out his research. For the psychologist, it is particularly tempting to accept the societal diagnosis, because most of the common psychological concepts refer to endopsychic processes. Like society, the psychologist may find it much more convenient to locate his concerns in the captive persons of the patients than in the less easily controlled and investigated processes that occur in the world outside.

To put research into "mental illness" on a scientific basis and to avoid the situation in which the researcher himself becomes one more arm of the societal reaction to nonconformity, it would seem that the medical model and its attendant psychiatric classifications would need to be eliminated from the program of research. Three areas particularly seem to require such reorientation. Those psychologists who seek the causes of nonconforming behavior should measure their dependent variable behaviorally and independently of the official societal reaction. Although there have been studies of "mental illness" in which the research has conceptually and operationally defined the dependent variable, the usual pattern is for the study to depend directly or indirectly (as in "known-group" validation) on the societal diagnosis.

A second research area is in the investigation of the micropolitical and social-psychological process of extrusion in small groups such as families, organizational factions, and neighborhood groups. Very little systematic information is now available on the conditions under which extrusion occurs and on the functions that it fulfills for the group.

A third and final area suggested by this discussion for systematic research is on the dynamics of decision-making in welfare and control agencies. The processes of information transmission, selective perception, and agency-client conflict in these agencies have received little attention from scientific investigators. One example of the type of study needed is an investigation of epidemiological differences in rates of mental illness in terms less of the incidence of disease than in variations in administrative process. A second example of organizational research would concern decision-making in treatment processes. A description of this type follows.

TYPIFICATION IN DIAGNOSIS

In the following discussion, I wish to indicate one particular avenue of research that would move outside the traditional research perspective in rehabilitation. The subject of this discussion is diagnostic, prognostic, and treatment stereotypes of officials and clients and the ways in which these influence treatment processes. Following Sudnow, I use the generic term, *normal cases*. The discussion begins with a review of Balint's (1957) concepts concerning doctor-patient relationships.

One of Balint's conclusions is that there is an apostolic function, that is, doctors in some ways function as apostles, seeking to proselytize their patients into having the kinds of diseases that the doctor thinks are conceivable in their cases (p. 216). It would be easy to accept Balint's statement concerning apostolic mission as academic hyperbole, which is used to make a subtle point concerning physical and psychiatric diagnosis. However, one can also take Balint's statement as literally true and talk about the kinds of organizations and the kinds of situations in which diagnostic stereotypes are used in classifying clientele and become the base for action.

The literal use of such stereotypes is apparent in Sudnow's "Normal Crimes" (1965). Making observations in the public defender's office in the court of a large city, he notes that the effective diagnostic unit for the public defender is the *typical* kind of crime: that is, crime typical for this city (the city that he describes) and this time in history. He describes burglary, child molestation, assault with a deadly weapon, and other crimes in terms of the folklore about these crimes that exists in the court in that particular city. To say that this is folklore is not to say that it is completely or even mostly inaccurate. The point that is made, however, is that the thinking of the public defender is in terms of these stereotypic crimes, and his questioning of the defendant is not so much an attempt to find the particular dimensions and aspects of the situation in which the defendant finds himself but almost entirely the extent to which this defendant seems to fit into the stereotyped category of criminal that exists in the court.

I will not attempt to repeat details of this article here. The point that is relevant is that these stereotypes are the functional units that are used by the public defender and, apparently, to a large extent, by the public prosecutor also in carrying out the business of the court. In this particular case, also, it should be noted that the aim of the public defender in using these stereotypes is not so much an attempt to get an acquittal but a reduction of sentence. This technique is therefore a way of maintaining a smooth-running operation of the court without gross violation of either the court's concept of punishment, on the one hand, or the defendant's rights, on the other.

It seems likely that such diagnostic stereotypes function in many kinds of treatment, control, and welfare agencies. As the functional units in which business gets done, it is important to note, however, that these diagnostic packages are of different importance in different kinds of organizations and situations. In the kind of situation that one may find, say, in the surgical ward of an outstanding hospital, one would assume that diagnostic stereotypes are used as preliminary hypotheses, which are retained or rejected on the basis of further investigation—that is, at one pole of the organizational continuum. At the other pole, in the kind of situation that Sudnow describes, these stereotypes are not only first hypotheses but also the final result of the investigation. That is, there is a tendency to accept these stereotyped descriptions with a very minimal attempt to see if they fit the particular case at hand. Later in this discussion, I state some propositions that relate the type of situation, the type of organization, and the functional importance of the diagnostic stereotypes.

The idea of "normal cases" would seem to offer an entering wedge for research in the most diverse kinds of agencies. In current medical practice, the dominant perspective is the "doctrine of specific etiology" (Dubos 1959). This perspective, largely an outgrowth of the successful application of the germ theory of disease, gives rise to the stance of "scientific medicine" in which the conceptual model of disease is a determinate system. The four basic components of this system are a single cause (usually a pathogen in the body), a basic lesion, uniform and invariant symptoms, and regularly recurring outcome, usually damage to the body or death if medical intervention is not forthcoming.

The model of disease in scientific medicine gives rise to "normal cases" in which diagnosis, prognosis, and treatment are somewhat standardized. (Thus, diabetes melitus is a disease in which the basic lesion is glucose intolerance, primary features are nutritional and metabolic disorders and susceptibility to infection, secondary features are retinopathy, coronary heart disease, renal disease, or neuropathy, and treatment is by routine insulin control.) An important component of this disease model is the application for treatment by the patient with complaints that are traceable to the disease. [Feinstein (1963) uses the term *lanthanic* for patients who have the disease but either do not have complaints or whose complaints do not result in application for treatment.] Cases in which the disease is present but the symptoms are not are obvious deviations from the "normal case" and cause difficulties in medical practice and research. Equally troublesome are causes in which the primary or secondary features of the disease are present but in which the basic lesion is absent. Meador (1965) has suggested, only half in jest, that such conditions be given specific medical status as "nondiseases."

The concept of *normal cases is* closely connected with the notion, in medicine, that physicians have of "What's going around." That is, in a normal practice, a physician is not exposed to all kinds of the most diverse diseases that are described in medical textbooks but only rather a small sample of diseases that come in repeatedly: colds, flu, appendicitis, nervous headaches, low back pain, etc.

Proportionately as the case load increases, or inversely as the amount of time that the physician has for each case, as the amount of interest he has, or as the amount of knowledge he has increases, one would expect that these diagnostic stereotypes would play an important role. Some of the atrocity tales of medical practice in armed services or in industry suggest the kinds of eventualities that can occur. For example, at the extreme, in some medical clinics for trainees in the army, virtually all treatments fall into one or two categories—aspirins for headaches and antihistamines for colds, and possibly a third category—a talk with a commanding officer for the residual category of malingerers.[2]

It is conceivable that the same kinds of conceptual packages would be used in other kinds of treatment, welfare, and control agencies. Surely in rehabilitation agencies, the conceptual units that the working staff uses cover only a rather limited number of contingencies of disability, placement possibilities, and client attitudes. The same minimal working concepts should be evident in such diverse areas as probation and parole, divorce cases, adoption cases, police handling of juveniles, and in the area of mental health.

Perhaps the most important characteristic of normal diagnoses, prognoses, and treatments is their validity. How accurate are the stereotypes that agency workers and patients use in considering their situations? One would guess that validity of stereotypes is related to their precision. Other things being equal, the more precise the stereotypes, the more ramified they are in the various characteristics of the client, the situation, and the community, the more accurate one would guess that they would be. Proposition 1, therefore, concerns simply the number of the different stereotypes that are used in an agency. One would guess that validity and precision are correlated:

Proposition 1: *The more numerous the stereotypes that are actually used in the agency, the more precise they will be, and the more precise they will be, the more valid they will be.*

Proposition 2 concerns the power of clients. Using the term *marginality* in the sense used by Krause, the more marginal the patients, the less numerous, precise, and valid the stereotypes will be (cited by Myers 1965):

Proposition 2: *The more the status of the client is inferior to and different from that of the staff, whether because of economic position, ethnicity, race, education, etc., the more inaccurate and final the normal cases will be.*

Proposition 3: *The less dependent the agent is upon the client's good will, the less precise and valid the stereotypes will be.*

In the situation of private practice, where the physician is dependent for remuneration upon the patient, one is more likely to find a situation as outlined by Balint (1957, p. 18), where decision concerning the patient's diagnosis becomes a matter of bargaining. This discussion qualifies Balint's formulation by suggesting that bargaining or negotiation is a characteristic of a medical service in which patients are powerful, such that the diagnostic stereotypes of the physician are confronted by the diagnostic stereotypes of the patient, and that the patient has some power to regulate the final diagnosis.

Proposition 4 relates to the body of knowledge in the agency or profession that is handling the clients. One would suspect that:

Proposition 4: *The more substantial or scientific the body of knowledge, the less important, the more valid, and the more accurate the conceptual packages.*

In areas of general medicine, for example, such as pneumonia and syphilis, the kind of stereotyping process discussed here is relatively unimportant. The same would be true in some areas of physical rehabilitation.

Proposition 5 relates the socialization of the staff member to his use of conceptual packages. One would assume that:

Proposition 5: *A fairly accurate index of socialization into an agency would be the degree to which a staff member uses the diagnostic packages that are prevalent in that agency.*

This proposition suggests a final proposition that is somewhat more complicated, relating effectiveness of a staff member in diagnosis or prognosis to his use of diagnostic stereotypes. One would guess that:

Proposition 6: *Effectiveness has a curvilinear relationship to knowledge and use of stereotypes.*

In the beginning, a new staff member would have only theory and little experience to guide him and would find that his handling of clients is time-consuming and his diagnoses tend to be inaccurate. As he learns the conceptual packages, he becomes more proficient and more rapid in his work, so that effectiveness increases. The crucial point comes after a point in time in which he has mastered the diagnostic packages, and the question becomes, Is his perceptiveness of client situations and placement opportunities going to remain at this stereotypic level, where it is certainly more effective than it was when he was a novice in the organization? Is it going to become frozen at this stereotypic level or is he going to go on to begin to use these stereotypes as hypotheses for guiding further investigation on his part? I would suggest that this is a crucial point in the career of any staff member in an agency, and the research that would tell us about this crisis would be most beneficial.[3]

Although carrying out research with normal cases could involve fairly complex procedures (e.g., in checking on the validity of diagnostic stereotypes in a series of cases), the beginning efforts in research could be fairly simple. One of the first questions I would want to ask in beginning a study of this kind would be something like, What kinds of cases do you see most of here in this agency?

With only a little elaboration, I believe such a question would elicit some of the standard stereotypes from most agency staff. Just describing the structure of the normal cases in an agency would be a major step in understanding how that organization functions.

A more ambitious program of research into diagnostic and prognostic treatment stereotypes would be to relate them in each case with the actual outcome of the case. An intermediate stage of research would be represented by any type of gaming study in which experienced, knowledgeable professionals would be assigned simulated cases given information that was found to be the prototypic information used in a given agency. A device for this purpose has been developed by Leslie Wilkins, as found in the appendix of his book on social deviance (1965, pp. 294–304). Wilkins calls this device an "information board." It contains a large number of items, say 50 items, in which the classification of information from a case history appears on separable index cards with titles of the information appearing on the visible edge of the cards. For example, in the work with probation officers that he did as a pilot study, the information board contained charge, complainant's account of incident, codefendant's account of incident, offender's account of incident, general appearance of the offender, sex and age of the offender, scholastic attainment, practical handling of problems by the offender, attitudes toward authority, and so on. In the various games that Wilkins had these probation trainees play, he allowed them to select several items from the possible list and then make a decision. With a little experimentation, it should not be difficult to devise diagnostic games with an information board that could be played by the staff of almost any kind of agency.

The two principal kinds of information needed in the proposed research would be, first, of the kind of dimensions of client condition or behavior that the staff actually uses in its day-to-day decision-making, whether these be blood pressure, race, continence, attitude toward authority, activity level, prior history of sexual propriety, and so on; and, second, the constellations of values of these dimensions into which the staff (and clients) combine these elements of information into "normal cases."

Conceptually, there remain a number of difficulties. In some ways, this kind of research is congenial to the approach anthropologists take toward the medical institutions of a small society: the approach to "folk medicine." Anthropological studies of folk medicine seek to describe the medical institutions of a society without accepting the underlying presuppositions of that society. In the same way, the approach to rehabilitation process by way of normal cases seeks to study the flow of business in an organization without accepting the presuppositions of the staff and clients involved. It should be remembered in this connection, however, that in many organizations there are at least two sets of folk involved, staff and clients, each possibly having vastly different sets of folk categories of illness or guilt, etc.

From the point of view of orderly conceptual formulation, none of the concepts used in this discussion (e.g., *diagnostic stereotypes, normal cases,* and *conceptual packages*) is particularly satisfactory. The concept of *stereotypes* implies more distortion than is intended and does not articulate very well with organizational structure.[4] *Normal cases* is a good enough general term but does not lead to a more detailed breakdown of subelements.[5] *Conceptual packages is* much too general a term. Perhaps the best set of concepts would be taken from role analysis. Normal cases imply a set of role expectations that articulate with the position of the perceiver in the organization. Diagnostic stereotypes in medicine, for example, may be construed as the counter-role variants that make up the physicians' role-set for patients. The concept of *role* seems somewhat static for this use and does not immediately suggest conceptual analogies for prognostic (role-futures?) or treatment stereotypes. Perhaps some of these difficulties can be removed through further discussion.

One way of conceptualizing the problem in a broader context is in terms of the *work system* in organizations. Often there is considerable difference between the official version of the work done in an organization and what actually gets done. The preceding discussion suggests that there may be a relatively small number of dimensions that determine the actual work system: the typifications previously described, the consensus on work rates (suggested by Howard Becker), and the precision and dependability with which work output is measured, for example. These dimensions provide the bare suggestions that the culture of the workplace may be considered to be any overdetermined, self-maintaining system and should therefore be studied as an analytical whole.

The purpose of these comments has been to formulate the kind of research that would avoid the undue emphasis on the individual and the physical as well as other presuppositions of the professionals who specialize in the rehabilitation process. This difference of viewpoint from those used in the agencies would likely cause some practical difficulties in carrying out research of this kind. Difficulties of a methodological and conceptual character have already been alluded to. Nevertheless, the program of research suggested here may provide a useful approach to a large number of problems in rehabilitation and medical organizations.

MENTAL ILLNESS AND SOCIAL STATUS

It would appear that the looseness of psychiatric theory and procedures, interacting with the attitudes of persons in the community, welfare, and control agencies, gives rise to a situation in which individualistic concepts, whether medical or psychological, can explain only part of the variation in the handling of the mentally ill. It has been suggested here that the serious student of regularities in our society may find it profitable to study "mental illness" in terms of "career contingencies" and social status.

Sociologically, a status is defined as a set of rights and duties. Although we tend to take the rights and duties of the ordinary citizen for granted, it becomes clear that there is an extensive set of rights and duties that define the status of the sane when we realize the rights that are abridged when a person is declared mentally incompetent (i.e., roughly speaking, when he is committed to a mental hospital). The following is a partial list of such rights:

Legal Areas Involving Competency
    1. Making a will (testamentary capacity)
    2. Making a contract deed, sale

3. Being responsible for a criminal act
4. Standing trial for a criminal charge
5. Being punished for a criminal act
6. Being married
7. Being divorced
8. Adopting a child
9. Being a fit parent
10. Suing and being sued
11. Receiving property
12. Holding property
13. Making a gift
14. Having a guardian, committee, or trustees
15. Being committed to a mental institution
16. Being discharged from a mental institution
17. Being paroled or put on probation
18. Being responsible for a tortious civil wrong
19. Being fit for military service
20. Being subject to discharge from the military service
21. Operating a vehicle
22. Giving a valid consent
23. Giving a binding release or waiver
24. Voting
25. Being a witness (testimonial capacity)
26. Being a judge or juror
27. Acting in a professional capacity, as a lawyer, teacher, physician
28. Acting in a public representative capacity, as a governor, legislator
29. Acting in a fiduciary capacity, as trustee, executor
30. Managing or participating in a business, as a director, stockholder
31. Receiving compensation for inability to work as a result of an injury.
    (Mezer and Rheingold 1962)

It should be understood that this list includes only those rights that are formally abrogated, either during or after hospitalization. Such a collection of abrogated rights points out that there is a distinct and separate status for the mentally ill in our society.

Throughout this chapter, there have been instances in which the mental patient has been compared with other disadvantaged persons of low social status. In this final section, it is argued that it is helpful to make a formal statement in which discussions of mental illness are translated to the language of social role and status; the social institution of insanity can be considered to be constituted by a "status line" between persons designated as sane and those designated to be mentally ill.

Most sociological concepts that have been developed to describe status lines refer to the norms that govern contact between races: the "color line." The structure of a color line, as formulated by Strong (1943) and others is built up around two statuses: the status of the in-group member and that of the out-group member.[6] Between these two statuses is the category of exception for persons assigned to neither group. Finally, completing the axis of statuses is the status ideal, which embodies the values of the in-group, and the negative status ideal, which embodies the vices. That is, the status ideals portray the in-group hero and villain, respectively. Corresponding to each of the five statuses is the appropriate role, which specifies the characteristics of persons occupying the status (see Figure 10.1).

Applied to the status line that separates deviants and nondeviants, this axis would contain the ideal status or hero of conformity to in-group values, the conventional conforming role, the categories of exception, which have neither deviant nor nondeviant status, the conventional deviant status, and the negative ideal, or supervillain.

Applied to the status separation between the sane and insane, the negative ideal would be the "raving lunatic" of heroic proportions and other such stereotypes that embody the most intense fears and aversions of the community. The status of the insane would be the conventional negative status, being roughly the status of the committed mental patient. The categories of exception would correspond to such conditions as "nervous breakdown," as used as a euphemism in popular parlance, and "temporary insanity," in which a person's behavior is excused without penalty.

The conventional conforming status would be that of the ordinary citizen whose sanity has not been called in question. What corresponds in our society to the status ideal on this axis of separation? In earlier societies, such a question would have been less difficult to answer, since most societies have held unambiguous and largely uncontested images of the virtuous man. In medieval Japan, for example, the image of the samurai would undoubtedly correspond to the status ideal. In our own earlier history, the members of the "elect" predestined to God's grace, would also fit this status. In contemporary society, however, religious authority no longer serves to give unquestioned legitimacy to the positive virtues, and the formulation of the role ideal is continuously in process.

It may be that the nearest that our society comes to a status ideal along the sane-insane axis is the concept of *positive mental health*. Jahoda (1958) reports no consensus among psychological experts on the criterion of positive mental health. The following six criteria are among those most prominent:

1. Attitudes toward one's self: self-esteem, correctness of self-conception, etc.
2. Growth, development, or self-actualization
3. Integration of the self
4. Autonomy; independence

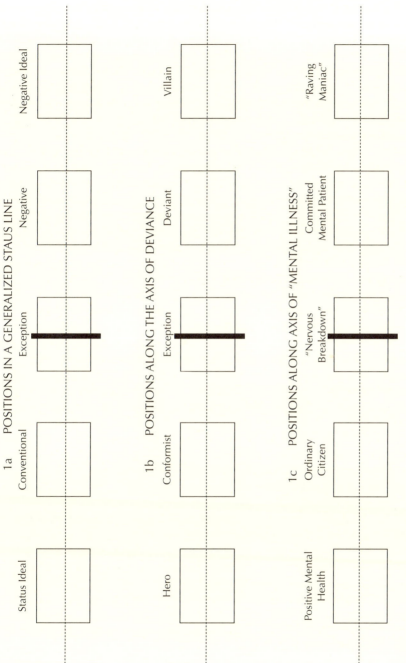

1a   POSITIONS IN A GENERALIZED STAUS LINE

Status Ideal   Conventional   Exception   Negative   Negative Ideal

1b   POSITIONS ALONG THE AXIS OF DEVIANCE

Hero   Conformist   Exception   Deviant   Villain

1c   POSITIONS ALONG AXIS OF "MENTAL ILLNESS"

Positive Mental Health   Ordinary Citizen   "Nervous Breakdown"   Committed Mental Patient   "Raving Maniac"

Figure 10.1.   Status lines.

5. Adequacy of perception of reality
6. Mastery of the environment

These disparate and conflicting criteria of mental health would appear to be little related to ordinary notions of health but rather formulations of what the various authors regard to be the highest values to which our society ought to aspire in shaping ourselves and our children. As such values, the concept of *positive mental health* comes very close to being what has been described as the status ideal.

Wallace's biocultural model of mental illness bears some resemblance to this model of the status line (1961). Wallace describes five *states* that make up the "theory" of mental illness held by the members of a society: Normalcy (N), Upset (U), Psychosis (P), In Treatment (T), and Innovative Personality (I). The sequences of states are presented in the following diagram:

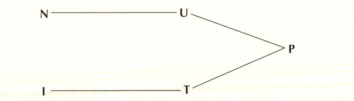

In the case where the Innovative Personality is equivalent to Normalcy, the diagram becomes:

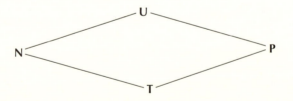

In this version, N corresponds to the conventional status, and P to the deviant status, with U and T representing the unlabeled and labeled phases of primary rule breaking, respectively. Both of these phases fall on or near the status line that separates the in-group and out-group.

There is one way in which the Wallace model is fundamentally different from the one presented here, however. His model is based on beliefs of members of the society, their "theories" of behavior, and is not directly connected with actual behavior. In the model of the status system discussed here, the positions in the system are actual social positions, each composed of a set of rights and duties, each recognized as legitimate social entities by the members of the society. Corresponding to the transfer mechanisms that Wallace posits (the mechanisms that explain to the satisfaction of the members of the society how the sick person moves from one state to another) would be the actual social procedures in the present model, the *rites de passage that* accomplish the transfer of the person from one status to another. Thus, Wallace's model complements the social system model, since it concerns the individual beliefs that accompany behavior. It would appear that both of the models are necessary to describe the system of behavior involved in the recognition and treatment of mental illness.

One of the most important characteristics of any status system is its permeability (i.e., the ease or difficulty of passage from one status to another). A status system that is impermeable is called a *caste system;* a status system that is permeable may be called a *class system.* Many of the reform programs that have been carried on in the last several decades in the mass media and more recently in the mental hospitals have been attempts to make the system more permeable, to desegregate first and then, after desegregation, to democratize the status of the mentally ill.

Needless to say, these programs have met with some outstanding successes: it is undoubtedly true that the typical mental patient today has a much better chance of passing back into his nondeviant status than he would have had 50 or even 25 years ago. It is also true, however, that the status system of insanity still has castelike aspects, as can be still seen on the back wards of most mental hospitals as well as in many other ways. It is also true that increasing permeability in such a status system means not only that those in the status of the insane can pass more easily into the sane status, but also that those in the sane status can pass more easily into that of the insane. It has been frequently remarked by planners or mental health services that such services appear to be bottomless pits; the more that are provided, the more demand there seems to be.

> An interesting, if somewhat unfortunate, consequence of the fact that social attitudes play such a big role in the definition of mental illness is that mental health education may be a two-edged sword. By teaching people to regard certain types of distress or behavioral oddities as illnesses rather than as normal reactions to life's stresses, harmless eccentricities, or moral weaknesses it may cause alarm and increase the demand for psychotherapy. This may explain the curious fact that the use of psychotherapy tends to keep pace with its availability. The greater the number of treatment facilities and the more widely they are known, the larger the number of persons seeking their help. Psychotherapy is the only form of treatment which, at least to some extent, appears to create the illness it treats. (Frank 1961, p. 67)

Increasing permeability could also mean, as Szasz has suggested, simply that more diverse kinds of problems—welfare, moral, political—are being funneled into psychiatric channels. In a thoughtful review of what he calls the "inflationary demand" for psychiatric services, Schofield (1964) makes the following observation:

> It is time for the leaders of the mental health movement to put their minds to . . . analysis of problems which psychiatry and psychology have tended to neglect: to criteria of mental health, to delimitation of the meanings and forms of mental illness, to specification of precisely what are and what are not *psychiatric* problems. It would be a positive contribution for mental health educators to develop ways of communicating to the public on such questions as: "When not to go to the psychiatrist"; or "What to do before you see a psychiatrist"; "What psychotherapy cannot do for you"; "Ten sources of helpful conversations"; "Problems which do not make you a 'Mental Case.'" (p. 147)

Both Frank and Schofield seem to be counseling the need for normalization in the face of the tendencies toward routine labeling in the ideology of the mental health movement.

These considerations pose policy problems, which, as such, are not the main focus of this discussion. We have sought in this book to provide a framework that would allow for a disciplined description of the way in which persons deemed mentally ill are handled in our society. It is not intended that this framework be accepted as a precise description of the social system that is operative in mental illness processes but only as a step toward more adequate theory and research. Such a framework may prove useful not only in research on mental illness but also in related areas of deviant behavior, such as crime and mental retardation. As has been mentioned before, race relations also would seem to have structures and dynamics similar to those outlined here.

One field, finally, that deserves mention in this connection is international relations. Perry (1957), in his formulation of "the role of the national," has begun the kind of conceptualization of the status dynamics between nations that has been discussed here for mental illness. Such formulations are badly needed in many areas of social science, since they promise to provide a bridge between social and individual processes. The integration of these two areas of research remains one of the principal tasks of social science. The theory presented here is intended as a step toward such integration.

* * * * *

This book outlines an approach to the study of mental illness that takes the motive forces out of the individual patient and puts them into the system constituted by the patient, other persons reacting to him, and the official agencies of control and treatment in the society. The theory and the evidence relevant to the truth or falsity of the theory are presented in the first part of the book. Acknowledging that the evidence is far from complete, both in amount and quality, the author concludes that the existing state of evidence favors this sociological theory, perhaps only slightly, relative to the alternative traditional theory based on the individual system model. Obviously, the author is predisposed to accept the theory and may not have been sufficiently impartial in his selection and evaluation of the evidence. Other investigators, more objective than the author, may review the state of evidence and come to a contrary conclusion. Perhaps it may be worthwhile if such a review were made, independently, assessing the state of evidence with respect to each of the propositions in Part I.

The same point may be made with respect to studies of decision-making in general medicine and psychiatry. Studies similar to these may be repeated in different settings by independent investigators to assess the validity and generality of the results reported here. Both the review of the state of evidence and the field studies repeating those reported here would likely be contributions to the developing sociology of mental illness.

A more valuable contribution may be made, however, if instead of seeking to repeat the assessment of the literature or the field studies reported here, other researchers sought to modify and refine the theory and research techniques discussed in this volume. The propositions in Part I, at their best, are very crude statements, lacking specificity and rigor. The nine propositions discussed represent a somewhat arbitrary selection from a larger number of propositions implicit in the theory. This theory, it would seem, should serve as a starting point for the development of a more complete and coherent set of propositions. This set, in turn, could lead to better research and further our understanding both of mental illness and of social processes that regulate conformity and deviance.

In future research informed by this theory, it would be desirable to increase not only the specificity but also the scope of the investigation. A large-scale study that tested many of the propositions simultaneously can easily be envisioned. One such study, for example, would be a longitudinal field study of residual rule-breakers that used an experimental design. In such a study, a survey would be used to locate rule-breakers who have not been labeled in the community. The rule-breakers would be divided into groups according to the amount and degree of their violations, with perhaps one group who repeatedly violates fundamental rules, at one extreme, and at the other, a group of persons who infrequently violates less important rules. Whatever the number and composition of these groups, each would be further divided at random into a labeled group and normalization group. That is, the rule-breakers in the labeled group would be exposed to the normal processes of recognition, definition, and treatment as mentally ill, and the denial group would be shielded from such processes. The effects of the labeling and normalization could then be systematically assessed over a period of time.

To carry out such a study properly, even with a relatively small sample of rule-breakers would require rather large amounts of money, time, and ingenuity. It would involve some taxing and delicate problems of ethics in research and of the responsibility of the researcher to his subjects and to the community. Nevertheless, if the position discussed here has any validity, if only in small part, the results of such a study could be enormously revealing. The likely conclusion of such a study would not be a clear verification or falsification of this theory but of indications of the conditions under which the social system determines case outcomes: the type of rule-breaker, community, psychiatric or other treatment, and situation in which the social system theory gives a fairly accurate picture of the sequence of events.

Future research aside, how successfully does the present discussion meet its proposed tasks: to formulate a purely sociological theory of chronic mental illness, to compare this theory with current alternative theories, and to judge the relative worth of these competing theories? Some shortcomings are obvious. The exclusion of the personal characteristics of the rule-breaker from the analysis, for example, probably limits the predictive power of the theory. To take just one characteristic: if there is a general trait of suggestibility, as is sometimes argued, this trait would figure prominently in the process of entering or not entering the role of the mentally ill. Contrary to the assumption made here, rule-breakers do vary in their personal characteristics: some have intensely held convictions, some do not; some are sophisticated about legal and medical procedures, and others are not; some are deferential to authority, and so on. These characteristics are probably important in determining how resistant a rule-breaker will be to entering the deviant role when it is offered. Many other dimensions that would qualify and augment the theory could also be pointed out.

As was noted in Chapter 1, however, the purpose of this discussion is not that of final explanation but of a starting point for systematic analysis. To evaluate the usefulness of the theory, the reader must ask two questions: First, how convincing is the analysis of careers of mental illness, which use gross social processes such as denial and labeling rather than the intricate intrapsychic mechanisms postulated in the medical model? Second, to what extent does the "clash of doctrines," to use Whitehead's (1962) phrase, which is developed here, illuminate the current controversy over policy, theory, and research in the area of mental illness? A definitive answer to these questions may be provided by future research. For the present, the reader must be guided by his own inclination and judgment.

Do the ideas offered in this book have any immediate implications for treatment and research? Here I will discuss two directions for the future. Both suggestions return to the idea of consilience (Wilson 1998), of integrating different disciplinary approaches toward an organic whole.

IMPLICATIONS OF THE EMOTIONAL/RELATIONAL
WORLD FOR TREATMENT AND RESEARCH

One direction for treatment would be to integrate the biological, social, and psychological elements that are needed in dealing with mental disorder. As pointed out in the first chapter, there are indications that all three spheres contribute to the causation and maintenance of mental disorder, although knowledge is still uncertain. How could some balance be introduced into the biopsychiatric approach that is now dominant?

A preliminary step toward integration would be to require that a *treatment plan* be developed for all patients before they can be given psychoactive drugs. Most of these drugs are being dispensed by physicians, who see many more patients than do psychiatrists. The requirement of a treatment plan would remind them that they should be dealing not only with biological elements.

The idea of a broad treatment plan is implied in a comment by Herman (1992), in the context of a narrower issue, the desirability of informed consent to the use of psychoactive drugs for PTSS (Post-Traumatic Stress Syndrome) victims:

> The informed consent of the patient may have as much to do with the outcome as the particular medication prescribed. If the patient is simply ordered to take medication to suppress symptoms, she is once again disempowered. If, on the contrary, she is offered medication as a tool to be used according to her best judgement, it can greatly enhance her sense of efficacy and control. Offering medication in this spirit also builds a cooperative therapeutic alliance. (Herman 1992, p. 161)

This idea seems to me applicable to all mental patients, not just those with PTSS. Herman's comment is closely related to Lazare's (1989) negotiated approach to treatment, already referred to in Chapter 1. In first eliciting a request from the patient, often a request for medication, Lazare's method sets up a negotiation with the patient that empowers her, as Herman's comment suggests. But it also opens up a whole range of other possible treatments, implying, at least, the idea of a treatment plan.

I recall an example of an approach to integrated treatment that I observed may years ago when I observed Aaron Lazare and John Stoeckle together interviewing new patients at Massachusetts General Hospital. John, who was director of primary care, dealt with the physical aspects, Aaron with the psychological and social aspects of the patient's care. Both were incredibly quick in sizing up the patient's situation, the whole interview ranging from only 15 to 30 minutes. Lazare's 5-minute bursts of psychotherapy gave a whole new meaning to the idea of brief psychotherapy.

The point is that requiring a treatment plan before administering drugs might help to remind physicians and psychiatrists of the need to deal with the whole patient and the patient's social environment, not just with their bodies. Such a requirement could lead to more training in the psychological and social aspects of mental disorder for physicians and psychiatrists.

For future directions in research on mental disorder, I recommend the further exploration of what I have called the emotional/relational world. One direction that may be needed is adding a case study dimension to randomized clinical trials (RCTs), as suggested in Chapter 1. There are methodological difficulties with case studies, but their strengths tend to compensate for the weaknesses in the quantitative methods used in RCTs (and vice versa). In particular, case studies can uncover some of the emotional/relational world of the patient and the patient's social environment. For case studies as an alternative to RCTs, see Jacobs and Cohen (1999).

As mentioned in Chapter 1, an exemplary study of the emotional/world of mental patients was conducted by Stanton and Schwartz (1954). By investigating communications between staff and between staff and patient, they showed that every instance of increase in symptoms could be linked to the social environment, usually covert disagreements about the patient among the staff.

The work of George Brown and others (Vaughn and Leff 1976) on Expressed Emotion (EE) can be seen as a continuation of the Stanton and Schwartz research direction. Brown developed a method for exploring the attitudes of the relatives who were the caretakers for ex-mental patients. The is now a sizable body of EE studies that consistently show a moderately high correlation between relapse and the attitudes of the caretaker toward the patient (hostility and emotional overinvolvement).

The EE studies represent a method that lies between qualitative studies and quantitative studies. On the one hand, verbatim texts are used as data. An audiotape of the relative's description of the ex-patient is coded for hostility and emotional overinvolvement, which bases the study directly in discourse, as in qualitative studies. On the other hand, these results are treated quantitatively, and involve an individual (the ex-patient's relative), rather than the social relationship between the ex-patient and the relative.

The next step in the EE studies might be to analyze the discourse between the ex-patient and the relative, in order to enter the emotional/relational world that is involved in recovery and in relapse. A single case study by Ryan (1993) explored this approach. The author (Hooley 1986) of a quantitative EE study was good enough to lend Ryan the audiotape of relative–ex-patient dialogue from one of her cases (this case involves marital dialogue: the ex patient is the husband).

Ryan's microanalysis of the dialogue strongly suggests that the couple are alienated in the form of isolation between them, and that much of their discourse is marked by what I have called an "interminable quarrel," the form of conflict caused by shame/anger spirals. Since Ryan's article is based on a single case, his results are only suggestive. But EE studies might take the next step in their development if they would include a dimension of comparative case studies like Ryan's single case.

I propose that exploration of the emotional/relational world, both in treatment and research, may lead to an explosion of our knowledge about the social and psychological elements in mental disorder. To this extent, such research could be a step toward integrating biological and social/psychological components in mental disorder.

NOTES

1.   It should be noted that neither Lemert nor Laing and Esterson *demonstrate* their hypotheses, since their techniques are not rigorously systematic. Their findings and similar findings by others, however, appear to constitute sufficiently weighty evidence to suggest the need for research that departs radically from conventional psychiatric assumptions.

2.   Cf. Roth (1962, pp. 46–56).

3.   C. Spaulding has suggested the proposition that typification practices in organizations are also a function of hierarchical position: the higher a person is in the hierarchy (and therefore the more removed from organizational routine), the less stereotyped are his typifications.

4.   D. Zimmerman called my attention to Schutz's term, *typifications.*

5.   M. Loeb suggested that "standard cases" would be preferable terminology.

6.   For an application to deviance of concepts drawn from race relations, see Goffman (1957, p. 508).

Appendix

Impact of the 1966 Edition on Legislative Change

In 1967 I was called on to testify before a subcommittee of the California Assembly that was investigating mental health policy. The chair of the committee, Jerome Waldie, was surprised and shocked by my testimony on commitment proceedings in Wisconsin. He subsequently read *Being Mentally Ill*, and encouraged his staff to do so also. Using my questions, his hearings confirmed in California my findings in Wisconsin. Documentation for this passage can be found in "The Dilemma of Mental Commitments in California: A Background Document," Assembly Interim Committee on Ways and Means (1967).

The chief of the subcommittee staff, Arthur Bolton, told me that my book was the "Bible" of the group that wrote the Lanterman-Petris Bill, which became the new mental health law for California, and later, for the rest of the United States. The new law made it much more difficult to keep patients in a hospital indefinitely. In the long run, it has put pressure on states to close down their large and remote mental hospitals, and to build community mental health facilities.

I should also note a significant deletion of a recommendation that I had made in the law that was finally passed. I had predicted that the new law would close or downsize many large mental hospitals. For this reason, I recommended that community mental health centers be opened, to provide treatment for the patients who would be released. Although this feature was

strongly supported by the subcommittee, it was opposed by the various medical associations lobbying in the Assembly, and by then Governor Reagan. It
was the deletion of this recommendation that released many untreated mentally ill persons onto the streets, and not just the new law.

The whole process of changing the law is documented in Bardach (1972).

References

Arieti, Silvano, and J. M. Meth. 1959. Rare, unclassifiable, collective and exotic psychotic syndromes. P. 547 in Silvano Arieti (ed.), *American Handbook of Psychiatry*, vol. 1. New York: Basic Books.

Atkinson, M., and J. Heritage. 1984. *Structures of Social Action*. Cambridge: Cambridge University Press.

Ayd, F. 1998. APA report, Part IV. *Psychiatric Times*, p. 28.

Bakwin, H. 1945. Pseudocia pediatricia. *New England Journal of Medicine* 232: 691–697.

Balint, M. 1957. *The Doctor, His Patient, and the Illness*. New York: International Universities Press.

Bardach, Eugene. 1972. *The Skill Factor in Politics: Reforming the California Mental Health Law*. Berkeley: University of California Press.

Becker, Howard S. 1963. *Outsiders*. New York: Free Press.

Bell, Quentin. 1967. *On Human Finery*. New York: Schocken.

Benedict, Ruth. 1946. *Patterns of Culture*. New York: Mentor.

Benjamins, J. 1950. Changes in performance in relation to influences upon self-conceptualization. *Journal of Abnormal and Social Psychology* 45:473–480.

Bennett, A. M. H. 1961. Sensory deprivation in aviation. Pp. 606–607 in P. Soloman et al. (eds.), *Sensory Deprivation*. Cambridge, MA: Harvard University Press.

Bennett, C. C. 1960. The drugs and I. Pp. 606–607 in L. Uhr and I. G. Miller (eds.), *Drugs and Behavior*. New York: Wiley.

Berger, Peter L., and Thomas Luckmann. 1966. *The Social Construction of Reality: A Treatise in the Sociology of Knowledge*. New York: Doubleday.

Berne, E. 1964. *Games People Play*. New York: Grove.

Blake, R. R., and J. S. Mouton. 1961. Conformity, resistance and conversion. Pp. 1–2 in I. A. Berg and B. M. Bass (eds.), *Conformity and Deviation*. New York: Harper.

Blau, Z. S. 1956. Changes in performance in relation to influences upon self-conceptualization. *Journal of Abnormal and Social Psychology* 45(July):473–480.

Bowen, M. 1978. *Family Therapy in Clinical Practice*. New York: J. Aronson.

Braithwaite, J. 1989. *Crime, Shame, and Reintegration*. Cambridge: Cambridge University Press.

Brauchi, J. T. and L. J. West. 1961. Sleep deprivation. *Journal of the American Medical Association* 171:11.

Breggin, Peter. 1991. *Toxic Psychiatry*. New York: St. Martin's.

Breggin, Peter. 1997. *Brain-Disabling Treatments in Psychiatry*. New York: Springer.

Breggin, Peter. 1998. *Talking Back to Ritalin*. Monroe, ME: Common Courage Press.

Brill, H., and B. Malzberg. 1950. Statistical Report Based on Arrest Record of 5,354 Ex-patients. New York State Mental Hospitals (available from the authors).

Brown, Laura S. 1994. *Subversive Dialogues: Theory in Feminist Therapy*. New York: Basic Books.

Bruner, J. 1983. *Child's Talk*. New York: Norton. Cain, A. C. 1964. On the meaning of "playing crazy" in borderline children. *Psychiatry* 27(August):278–289.

Caudill, W., F. C. Redlich, H. R. Gilmore, and E. B. Brody. 1952. Social structure and interaction process on a psychiatric ward. *American Journal of Orthopsychiatry* 22(April):314–334.

Chernoff, H., and L. E. Moses. 1959. *Elementary Decision Theory*. New York: Wiley.

Clausen, J. A., and M. R. Yarrow. 1955. Paths to the mental hospital. *Journal of Social Issues* 11(December):2532.

Cohen, David. 1997. A critique of the use of neuroleptic drugs in psychiatry. In Seymour Fisher and Roger Greenberg (eds.), *From Placebo to Panacea: Putting Psychiatric Drugs to the Test*. New York: Wiley.

Coleman, J. V. 1964. Social factors influencing the development and containment of psychiatric symptoms. Paper presented to the First International Congress of Social Psychiatry, London, August.

Cooley, C. H. 1922. *Human Nature and the Social Order*. New York: Scribners.

Cumming, E., and Cumming, J. 1957. *Closed Ranks*. Cambridge, MA: Harvard University Press.

Darley, W. 1959. What is the next step in prevention medicine? *Association of Teachers Preventive Medicine Newsletter* 6.

Dawber, T. R., F. E. Moore, and G. V. Mann. 1957. Coronary heart disease in the Framingham Study, Part 2. *American Journal of Public Health* 47(April):4–24.

DeGrandpre, Richard. 1999. *Ritalin Nation*. New York: Norton.

Diller, Lawrence. 1998. *Running on Ritalin*. New York: Bantam.

Dubos, Rene. 1961. *Mirage of Health*. Garden City, NY: Doubleday-Anchor.

Durkheim, Emile. [1895] 1938. *The Rules of Sociological Method*. New York: Free Press.

Durkheim, Emile. 1915. *The Elementary Forms of the Religious Life*. Translated by Joseph Ward Swain. New York: Free Press.

Durkheim, Emile. 1963. Sociology and philosophy. In George Simpson (ed.), *Emile Durkheim*. New York: Thomas Y. Crowell.

Eichorn, R. L., and R. M. Andersen. 1962. Changes in personal adjustment to perceived and medically established heart disease: A panel study. Paper presented to American Sociological Association Annual Meeting, Washington, D.C.

Elias, Norbert. 1978. *The Civilizing Process*, vol. 1. New York: Vintage.

Elias, Norbert. 1982. *The Civilizing Process*, vol. 2. New York: Vintage.

Ellis, A. 1945. The sexual psychology of human hermaphrodites. *Psychosomatic Medicine* 7(March):108–125.

Erikson, Kai T. 1957. Patient role and social uncertainty—A dilemma of the mentally ill. *Psychiatry* 20:263–274.

Everson, S. A., Goldberg, D. E., and Kaplan, G. 1996. Hopelessness and risk of mortality. *Psychosomatic Medicine* 58:112–121.

Eysenck, Hans J. 1959. Learning theory and behavior therapy. *Journal of Mental Science* 105:61–75.

Feinstein, A. R. 1963. Boolean algebra and clinical taxonomy. *New England Journal of Medicine* 269(October):929–938.

Fenichel, O. 1945. *The Psychoanalytic Theory of Neurosis.* New York: Norton.

Fenwick, M. 1948. *Vogue's Book of Etiquette.* New York: Simon and Schuster.

Fisher, Seymour and Roger Greenberg (eds.). 1997. *From Placebo to Panacea.* New York: Wiley.

Fogelson, R. D. 1965. Psychological theories of windigo "sychosis" and a preliminary application of a models approach. Pp. 74–99 in M. E. Spiro (ed.), *Context and Meaning in Cultural Anthropology.* New York: Free Press.

Frank, Jerome D. 1961. *Persuasion and Healing.* Baltimore: Johns Hopkins University Press.

Friedman, Neil. 1967. *The Social Nature of Psychological Research: The Psychological Experiment as Social Interaction.* New York: Basic Books.

Gardiner-Hill, H. 1958. *Clinical Involvements.* London: Butterworth.

Garfinkel, H. 1956. Conditions of successful degradation ceremonies. *American Journal of Sociology* 61(March):420–424.

Garfinkel, H. 1964. Studies of the routine grounds of everyday activities. *Social Problems* 11(Winter):225–250.

Garland, L. H. 1959. Studies on the accuracy of diagnostic procedures. *American Journal of Roentgenology, Radium Therapy, and Nuclear Medicine* 82:25–38.

Gibbs, Jack. 1972. Issues in defining deviant behavior. Pp. 39–68 in Robert A. Scott and Jack D. Douglas (eds.), *Theoretical Perspectives on Deviance.* New York: Basic Books.

Gill, Merton, Robert Newman, and Friedrich Redlich. 1954. *The Initial Interview in Psychiatric Practice.* New York: International Universities Press.

Glass, A. J. 1953. Psychotherapy in the combat zone. In *Symposium on Stress.* Washington, DC: Army Medical Service Graduate School.

Goffman, E. 1957. Some dimensions of the problem. In Milton Greenblatt, D. J. Levinson, and R. H. Williams (eds.), *The Patient and the Mental Hospital.* Glencoe, IL: Free Press.

Goffman, E. 1959. *Asylums.* New York: Doubleday-Anchor.

Goffman, E. 1963. *Stigma.* Englewood Cliffs, NJ: Prentice-Hall.

Goffman, E. 1964. *Behavior in Public Place.* New York: Free Press.

Goffman, E. 1967. *Interaction Ritual.* New York: Anchor.

Gottschalk, L., C. Wingert, and G. Gleser. 1969. *Manual of Instruction for Using the Gottschalk-Gleser Content Analysis Scales.* Berkeley: University of California Press.

Gove, Walter (ed.). 1980. *Labeling Deviant Behavior.* Newbury Park, CA: Sage.

Gove, Walter (ed.). 1982. *Deviance and Mental Illness.* Newbury Park, CA: Sage.

Grob, Gerald. 1998. Psychiatry's Holy Grail: The search for the mechanisms of mental disease. *Bulletin of the History of Medicine* 72:189–219.

Haley, Jay. 1959. Control in psychoanalytic psychotherapy. Pp. 48–65 in *Progress in Psychotherapy,* vol. 4. New York: Grune and Stratton.

Haley, Jay. 1969. *The Power Tactics of Jesus Christ and Other Essays.* New York: Grossman.

Harrington, Ann (ed.). 1997. *The Placebo Effect.* Cambridge, MA: Harvard University Press.

Hastings, D. W. 1958. Follow-up results in psychiatric illness. *American Journal of Psychiatry* 114:1057–1066.

Hayward, M. L., and J. E. Taylor. 1956. A schizophrenic patient describes the action of intensive psychotherapy. *Psychiatric Quarterly* 30:211.

Healy, David. 1997. *The Antidepressant Era.* Cambridge, MA: Harvard University Press.

Herbert, C. C. 1961. Life-influencing interactions. In A. Simon et al. (eds.), *The Physiology of the Emotions.* Springfield, IL: Charles C. Thomas.

Herman, Judith. 1992. *Trauma and Recovery.* New York: Basic Books.

Heron, W. 1961. Cognitive and physiological effects of perceptual isolation. P. 817 in P. Solomon et al. (eds.), *Sensory Deprivation.* Cambridge, MA: Harvard University Press.

Hill, A. B. 1960. *Controlled Clinical Trials.* Springfield, IL: Charles C. Thomas.

Hochschild, Arlie. 1979. Emotion work, feeling rules, and social structure. *American Journal of Sociology* 85:551–575.

Hofstadter, D. 1975. *Goedel, Escher, Bach.* New York: Vintage.

Hollingshead, August B., and Frederich C. Redlich. 1958. *Social Class and Mental Illness.* New York: Wiley.

Hooley, Jill. 1986. Expressed emotion and depression: Interactions between patients and high- versus low-expressed emotion spouses. *Journal of Abnormal Psychology* 95:237–246.

Horowitz, M. 1981. Self-righteous rage. *Archives of General Psychiatry* 38:(November):1233–1238.

Ilg, F. L. and L. B. Ames. 1960. *Child Behavior.* New York: Dell.

Jacobs, David, and David Cohen. 1999. What is really known about psychological alternations produced by psychiatric drugs? *International Journal of Risk and Safety in Medicine* 12:(in press).

Jahoda, M. 1958. *Current Concepts of Positive Mental Health.* New York: Basic Books.

Kardiner, A., and H. Spiegal. 1947. *War Stress and Neurotic Illness.* New York: Hoeber.

Kellam, S. G., and J. B. Chassan. 1962. Social context and symptom fluctuation. *Psychiatry* 25:370–381.

Kelly, H., Berscheid, E., Christenson, A., Harvey, J., Huston, T., Levenger, G., McClintock, E., Peplau, L., and D. Peterson. 1983. *Close Relationships.* New York: W. H. Freeman.

Kinsey, A. C., W. B. Pomeroy, and C. E. Martin. 1948. *Sexual Behavior in the Human Male.* Philadelphia and London. W. B. Saunders.

Kirk, Stuart, and Herb Kutchins. 1992. *The Selling of DSM: The Rhetoric of Science in Psychiatry.* Hawthorne, NY: Aldine de Gruyter.

Klapp, Orin. 1962. *Heroes, Villains, and Fools.* Englewood Cliffs, NJ: Prentice-Hall.

Kohut, H. E. 1971. Thoughts on narcissism and narcissistic Rage. *The Search for the Self.* New York: International Universities Press.

Koos, E. L. 1954. *The Health of Regionville.* New York: Columbia University Press.

Kuhn, T. 1962. *The Structure of Scientific Revolutions.* Chicago: University of Chicago Press.

Kutchins, Herb, and Stuart Kirk. 1997. *Making Us Crazy.* New York: Free Press.

Labov, W., and D. Fanshel. 1977. *Therapeutic Discourse.* New York: Academic Press.

Laing, Ronald D. 1967. *The Politics of Experience,* New York: Ballantine.

Laing, Ronald D., and Aaron Esterson. 1964. *Sanity, Madness and the Family.* London: Tavistock.

Lancetot, Krista, et al. 1998. Efficacy and safety of neuroleptics in behavioral disorders associated with dementia. *Journal of Clinical Psychiatry* 59(10):550–561.

Lazare, Aaron. 1989. *Outpatient Psychiatry: Diagnosis and Treatment.* Baltimore: Williams and Witkin.

Ledley, R. S., and L. B. Lusted. 1959. Reasoning foundations of medical diagnosis. *Science* 130:9–21.

Leighton, D. C., et al. 1963. *The Character of Danger.* New York: Basic Books.

Lemert, E. M. 1951. *Social Pathology.* New York: McGraw-Hill.

Lemert, E. M. 1962. Paranoia and the dynamics of exclusion. *Sociometry* 25 (March): 220.

Lerman, Hannah. 1996. *Pigeonholing Women's Misery: A History and Critical Diagnosis of the Psychodiagnosis of Women in the Twentieth Century.* New York: Basic Books.

Lewis, H. 1971. *Shame and Guilt in Neurosis.* New York: International Universities Press.

Lewis, H. 1976. *Psychic War in Men and Women.* New York: New York University Press.

Lewis, H. 1979. Using content analysis to explore shame and guilt in neurosis. In L. Gottschalk (ed.), *The Content Analysis of Verbal behavior.* New York: Halstead.

Lewis, H. 1981a. *Freud and Modern Psychology. Volume 1: The Emotional Basis of Mental Illness.* New York: Plenum.

Lewis, H. 1981b. *Freud and Modern Psychology. Volume 2: The Emotional Basis of Human Behavior.* New York: Plenum.

Lewis, Jerry M. 1998. For better or worse: Interpersonal relationships and individual outcome. *American Journal of Psychiatry* 155:582–589.

Lieberman, S. 1956. The effect of changes in roles on the attitudes of role occupants. *Human Relations* 9:385–402.

Linden, M. 1964. Comment. Presented at the First International Congress of Social Psychiatry, London, August. *Sociology* 78(November):684–686.

Link, Bruce, and Cullen, Francis. 1990. The labeling theory of mental disorder: a review of the evidence. *Research in Community and Mental Health* 6:75–105.

Link, Bruce, Howard Andrews, and F. Cullen. 1992. The violent and illegal behavior of mental patients reconsidered. *American Sociological Review* 57:275–292.

Link, Bruce, Mirotznik, J., and Cullen, F. 1991. The effectiveness of stigma coping orientations: Can negative consequences of mental illness be avoided? *Journal of Health and Social Behavior* 32:302–320.

Link, Bruce, et al. 1997. On stigma and its consequences: Evidence from a longitudinal study. *Journal of Health and Social Behavior* 38:177–190.

Lunbeck, Elizabeth. 1994. *The Psychiatric Persuasion.* Princeton, NJ: Princeton University Press.

Mann, J. H. 1956. Experimental evaluations in role playing. *Psychological Bulletin.* 53:227–234.

Marx, Karl. 1906. *Capital.* New York: Modern Library.

Mead, G. H. 1934. *Mind, Self, and Society.* Chicago: University of Chicago Press.

Meador, C. K. 1965. The art and science of nondisease. *New England Journal of Medicine* 272(January):92–95.

Mechanic, David. 1963. One-sided analysis versus the eclectic approach. P. 167 in H. I. Leavitt (ed.), *The Social Science of Organizations.* Englewood Cliffs, NJ: Prentice-Hall.

Mechanic, David. 1999. *Mental Health and Social Policy.* Needham Heights, MA: Allyn and Bacon.

Mezer, R. R., and P. D. Rheingold. 1962. Mental capacity and incompetency: A psycho-legal problem. *American Journal of Psychiatry* 118:827–831.

Mirowsky, John. 1990. Subjective boundaries and combinations in psychiatric diagnoses. *Journal of Mind and Behavior* 11:407–424.

Myers, J. K. 1965. Consequences and prognoses of disability. Paper presented at the Conference on Sociological Theory, Research and Rehabilitation, Carmel, California, March.

Newman, Donald J. 1966. *Conviction: The Determination of Guilt or Innocence without Trial.* Boston: Little Brown.

Neyman, J. 1950. *First Course in Probability and Statistics.* New York: Holt.

Nietzsche, F. [1887] 1967. *On the Genealogy of Morals.* New York: Vintage.

Nunnally, J. C., Jr. 1961. *Popular Conceptions of Mental Health.* New York: Holt, Rinehart and Winston.

Parsons, T. 1950. Illness and the role of the physician. *American Journal of Orthopsychiatry* 21:452–460.

Pasamanick, B. 1963. A survey of mental disease in an urban population. IV: An approach to total prevalence rates. *Archives of General Psychiatry* 5 (August): 151–155.

Peirce, C. S. [1896–1908] 1955. Abduction and induction. Pp. 150–156 in J. Buchler (ed.), *Philosophical Writings of Peirce.* New York: Dover.

Perry, S. E. 1957. Notes on the role of the national. *Conflict Resolution* I(December):346–363.

Phillips, D. L. 1963. Rejection: A possible consequence of seeking help for mental disorder. *American Sociological Review* 28(December):963–973.

Pittenger, R., C. Hockett, and J. Danehy. 1960. *The First Five Minutes.* Ithaca, NY: Paul Martineau.

Plunkett, R. J., and J. E. Gordon. 1960. *Epidemiology and Mental Illness.* New York: Basic Books.

Porter, Roy. 1990. *A Social History of Madness.* New York: E. P. Dutton.

Porterfield, A. L. 1946. *Youth in Trouble.* Fort Worth, TX: Lee Potishman Foundation.

Ratner, H. 1962. Medicine. *Interviews on the American Character.* Santa Barbara, CA: Center for the Study of Democratic Institutions.

Rautaharju, P. M., M. J. Korvonen, and A. Keys. 1961. The frequency of arteriosclerotic and hypertensive heart disease in ostensibly healthy working populations in Finland. *Journal of Chronic Diseases* 13:426–438.

Retzinger, S. 1989. A theory of mental illness: Integrating social and emotional aspects. *Psychiatry,* 52 (3):325–335.

Rogler, L. H., and August B. Hollingshead. 1965. *Trapped: Families and Schizophrenia*. New York: Wiley.

Rosenthal, Robert. 1966. *Experimenter Effects in Behavioral Research*. New York: Appleton-Century Crofts.

Rosenzweig, N. 1959. Sensory deprivation and schizophrenia: Some clinical and theoretical similarities. *American Journal of Psychiatry* 116:326.

Ross, Collin, and Alvin Pam. 1995. *Pseudoscience in Biological Psychiatry: Blaming the Body*. New York: Wiley

Roth, Julius A. 1963. *Timetables: Structuring the Passage of Time in Hospital Treatment and Other Careers*. Indianapolis.: Bobbs-Merrill.

Roth, Philip. 1962. Novotny's pain. *New York* (October 27):46–56.

Ryan, Michael. 1993. Shame and expressed emotion: A case study. *Sociological Perspectives* 36:167–183.

Sachar, Edward J. 1963. Behavioral science and criminal law. *Scientific American* 209: 39–45.

Sacks, H. 1966. *The Search for Help: No One to Turn To*. Ph.D dissertation, University of California, Berkeley, University Microfilms.

Sacks, H., E. Schegloff, and G. Jefferson. 1974. A simplist systematics for the organization of turn-taking in conversation. *Language* 50, 696–735.

Sadow, L., and A. Suslick. 1961. Simulation of a previous psychotic state. *AMA Archives of General Psychiatry* 4(May):452–458.

Saunders, L. 1954. *Cultural Differences and Medical Care*. New York: Russell Sage Foundation.

Scheff, Thomas J. 1966. Hospitalization of the mentally ill in Italy, England and the United States. *Yearbook of the American Philosophical Society*. Philadelphia: American Philosophical Society.

Scheff, Thomas J. [1966] 1984. *Being Mentally Ill,* 2nd edition. Chicago: Aldine.

Scheff, Thomas J. 1979. *Catharsis in Healing, Ritual and Drama*. Berkeley: University of California Press.

Scheff, Thomas J. 1984. The taboo on coarse emotions. *Review of Personality and Social Psychology* 5:146–169.

Scheff, Thomas J. 1986. Microlinguistics: A theory of social action. *Sociological Theory* 4(1):71–83.

Scheff, Thomas J. 1987. The shame-rage spiral: case study of an interminable quarrel. In H. B. Lewis (ed.), *The Role of Shame in Symptom Formation*. Hillsdale, NJ: Erlbaum Associates.

Scheff, Thomas J. 1989. Emotions and understanding: Toward a theory and method. In S. Wapner (ed.), *Emotions in Ideal Human Development*. Hillsdale, NJ: Erlbaum Associates.

Scheff, Thomas J. 1990. *Microsociology: Discourse, Emotion and Social Structure*. Chicago: University of Chicago Press.

Scheff, Thomas J. 1994. *Bloody Revenge: Emotions, Nationalism, and War*. Boulder, CO: Westview.

Scheff, Thomas J. 1997. *Emotions, Social Bonds, and Human Reality: Part/Whole Analysis*. Cambridge: Cambridge University Press.

Scheff, T., and Bushnell, D. 1984. Cognitive and emotional components in anorexia: re-analysis of a classic case. *Psychiatry* 52:148–160.

Scheff, T., and Retzinger, S. 1991. *Emotions and Violence*. Lexington, MA: Lexington.

Scheler, M. [1912] 1961. *Resentment.* Glencoe, IL: Free Press.

Schelling, Thomas C. 1963. *The Strategy of Conflict.* New York: Oxford University Press.

Schofield, W. 1964. *Psychotherapy: The Purchase of Friendship.* Englewood Cliffs, NJ: Prentice-Hall.

Schutz, Alfred. 1962. *The Problem of Social Reality: Collected Papers 1.* The Hague: Martinus Nijhoff.

Schwartz, J., and G. L. Baum. 1957. The history of histoplasmosis. *New England Journal of Medicine* 256:253–258.

Scott, W. A. 1958. Research definitions of mental health and mental illness. *Psychological Bulletin 55* (January):29–45.

Settle, Edmund. 1998. Anti-depressant drugs: disturbing and potentially dangerous adverse effects. *Journal of Clinical Psychology* 59:Supplement 16.

Shapiro, Arthur K., and Elaine Shapiro. 1997. *The Powerful Placebo.* Baltimore: Johns Hopkins University Press.

Shibutani, T. 1959. *Society and Personality.* Englewood Cliffs, NJ: Prentice-Hall.

Srole, L., et al. 1962. *Mental Health in the Metropolis.* New York: McGraw-Hill.

Stanton, Alfred, and Morris Schwartz. 1954. *The Mental Hospital.* New York: Basic Books

Steiner, G. 1975. *After Babel.* London: Oxford University Press.

Stern, D. 1985. *The Interpersonal World of the Child.* New York: Basic Books.

Stern, D., L. Hofer, W. Haft, and J. Dore. 1984. Affect attunement: The sharing of feeling starts between mother and infant. In T. Field and N. Fox (eds.), *Social Perception in Early Infancy.* New York: Elsevier.

Stokes, J., and T. R. Dawber. 1959. The "silent coronary": The frequency and clinical characteristics of unrecognized myocardial infarction in the Framingham Study. *Annals of Internal Medicine* 50:1359–1369.

Strauss, Anselm, et al. 1963. The hospital and its negotiated order. Pp. 147–169 in Eliot Freidson (ed.), *The Hospital in Modern Society.* New York: Free Press.

Strauss, John. 1979. Do psychiatric patients fit their diagnosis? *Journal of Nervous and Mental Disease* 167:105–113.

Strong, S. M. 1943. Social types in a minority group. *American Journal of Sociology* 48(March):563–573.

Sudnow, David. 1965. Normal crimes: Sociological features of the penal code in a public defender's office. *Social Problems* 12(Winter):255–276.

Szasz, T. S. 1960. The myth of mental illness. *American Psychologist* 15(February): 113–118.

Szasz, T. S. 1961. *The Myth of Mental Illness.* New York: Hoeber-Harper.

Tavris, Carol. 1992. *The Mismeasure of Women.* New York: Simon and Schuster.

Thase, Michael, and David Kupfer. 1996. Recent developments in the pharmacotherapy of mood disorders. *Journal of Consulting and Clinical Psychology* 64: 646–659.

Thoits, P. 1985. Self-labeling processes in mental illness: the role of emotional deviance. *American Journal of Sociology* 91:221–248.

Tienari, Pekka, and Lyman Wynne. 1994. Adoption Studies of Schizophrenia. *Annals of Medicine* 26:233–237.

Traver, Robert. 1958. *Anatomy of a Murder.* New York: St. Martin's.

Tronick, E. Z., M. Ricks, and J. Cohn. 1982. Maternal and infant affect exchange: Patterns of adaption. In T. Field and A. Fogel (eds.), *Emotion and Early Interaction.* Hillsdale, NJ: Erlbaum Associates.

Trussel, R. E., J. Ehrlich, and M. Morehead. 1962. *The Quantity, Quality and Costs of Medical and Hospital Care Secured by a Sample of Teamster Families in the New York Area.* New York: Columbia University School of Public Health and Administrative Medicine.

Tucker, Gary. 1998. Putting DSM-IV in perspective. *American Journal of Psychiatry* 155:159–161.

Ullman, L. P., and L. Krasner. 1965. *Case Studies in Behavior Modification.* New York: Holt, Rinehart and Winston

Vaihinger, H. 1924. *The Philosophy of "as if."* London: Kegan Paul.

Valenstein, Elliot. 1998. *Blaming the Brain.* New York: Free Press.

Vaughn, C. E. and J. P. Leff. 1976. The influence of family and social factors on the course of psychiatric illness. *British Journal of Psychiatry* 125:157–165.

Vogel, E., and N. Bell. 1961. The emotionally disturbed child as the family scapegoat. Pp. 382–397 in N. W. Bell and E. F. Vogel (eds.), *A Modern Introduction to the Family.* London: Routledge and Kegan Paul.

Walker, Sydney. 1998. *The Hyperactivity Hoax.* New York: St. Martin's.

Wallace, Anthony F. C. 1961. Mental illness, biology and culture. Pp. 255–295 in Francis L. K. Hsu (ed.), *Psychological Anthropology.* Homewood, IL: Dorsey.

Wallerstein, J. S., and C. J. Wyle. 1947. Our law-abiding lawbreakers. *Probation* 25: 107–112.

Warner, W. L. 1958. *A Black Civilization.* New York: Harper.

Warren, J. V., and J. Wolter. 1954. Symptoms and diseases induced by the physician. *General Practitioner* 9:77–84.

Watzlawick, P., J. H. Beavin, and D. Jackson. 1967. *The Pragmatics of Human Communication.* New York: Norton.

Webb, Eugene J., Donald T. Campbell, Richard D. Schwartz, and Lee Sechrest. 1966. *Unobtrusive Measures: Nonreactive Research in Social Science.* Chicago: Rand-McNally.

Weber, M. 1949. *The Methodology of the Social Sciences* New York: Free Press.

Whitehead, Alfred N. 1962. *Science and the Modern World.* New York: Macmillan.

Wilkins, Leslie T. 1965. *Social Deviance: Social Policy, Action and Research.* Englewood Cliffs, NJ: Prentice-Hall.

Wilson, E. O. 1998. *Consilience: The Unity of Knowledge.* New York: Knopf.

Winograd, T. 1984. Computer software for working with language. *Scientific American* 251:130–145.

Yap, P. M. 1951. Mental diseases peculiar to certain cultures: A survey of comparative psychiatry. *Journal of Mental Science* 97(April):313–327.

Yarrow, M. R., et al. 1955. The psychological meaning of mental illness in the family. *Journal of Social Issues* 11(December):12–24.

Index